THE MUSCLES

Words in *italics* in the main
text (*or in* Roman *type in
the captions*) are explained
in the Index and glossary at
the end of the book.

A Cherrytree Book

Adapted by A S Publishing
from EL MÚSCULO ÓRGANO DE LA FUERZA
by Victoria Ávila
illustrated by Antonio Muñoz Tenllado
© Parramón Ediciones, S.A. – 1994

This edition first published 1995
by Cherrytree Press Ltd
a subsidiary of
The Chivers Company Ltd
Windsor Bridge Road
Bath, Avon BA2 3AX

© Cherrytree Press Ltd 1995

British Library Cataloguing in Publication Data

The Muscles. – (Invisible World Series)
  I. Halton, Frances II. Series
  611.71

  ISBN 0-7451-5258-9

Typeset by Dorchester Typesetting Group Ltd, Dorset
Printed in Spain

All rights reserved. No part of this publication may be
reproduced, stored in a retrieval system, or transmitted, in
any form or by any means without the prior permission in
writing of the publisher, nor be otherwise circulated in any
form of binding or cover other than that in which it is
published and without a similar condition including this
condition being imposed on the subsequent purchaser.

INVISIBLE WORLD

THE MUSCLES

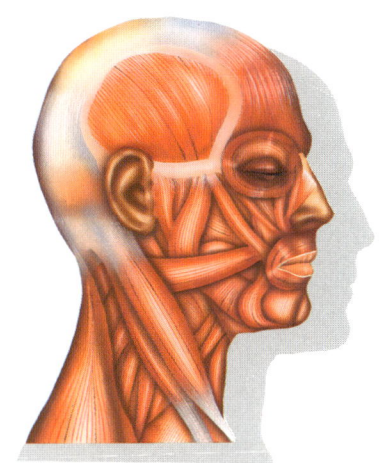

Edited by
Frances Halton

CHERRYTREE BOOKS

THE MUSCLES

Moving parts

Every movement of our bodies is controlled by our muscles. Even when we seem to be quite still our muscles are at work; they are controlling breathing, *digestion*, the beating of the *heart* and the circulation of blood around the body. Other muscles are holding the bones of our bodies in position. There are over 600 named muscles in the human body.

When you want to move your hand, your brain sends signals to the muscles involved in moving it and these carry out your orders. Muscles such as this, which we can control, are known as *voluntary muscles* and they make up about 40 per cent of total body weight. They are all made up of bundles of special muscle cells, or *muscle fibres*, and they work by contracting and relaxing. Some of them are very big, such as the *deltoid* muscles that help move our shoulders. Others, like those that move our eyes, are only a few millimetres long. Some make powerful movements and others control tiny, delicate actions.

Other muscles in the body work and are regulated without our being aware of it – the muscles that move the food along the *digestive tract*, for example. These are known as *involuntary muscles*, and they are able to contract and relax rhythmically without tiring.

The most important muscle of all is the *cardiac muscle* which makes up the heart, and beats steadily throughout our life. We have no conscious control over it.

When we talk about the muscular system, we normally refer to the voluntary muscles which, together with bones and joints, move our bodies. These diagrams show some of the most important voluntary muscles – others are hidden in deeper layers.

The oesophagus *is the tube which carries food from the pharynx at the back of the mouth down to the stomach.* It is about 25 centimetres long. Its walls contain layers of smooth (involuntary) muscle. They contract behind the food we swallow, and relax in front of it, propelling it along. This movement is known as a peristaltic wave. *We cannot control the movements of smooth muscle – this is done by unconscious nerve signals from the brain and in some cases by hormones.*

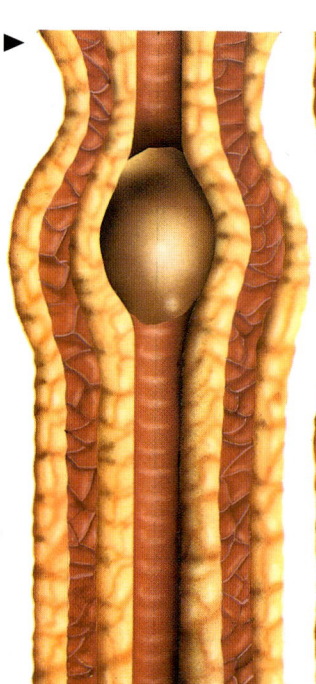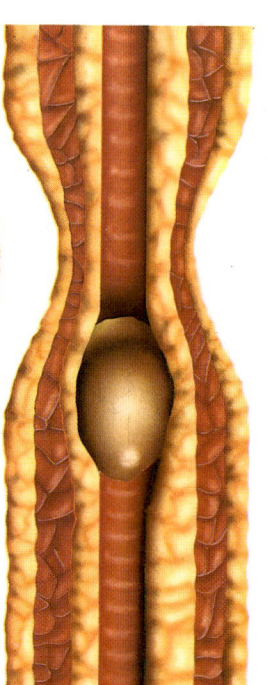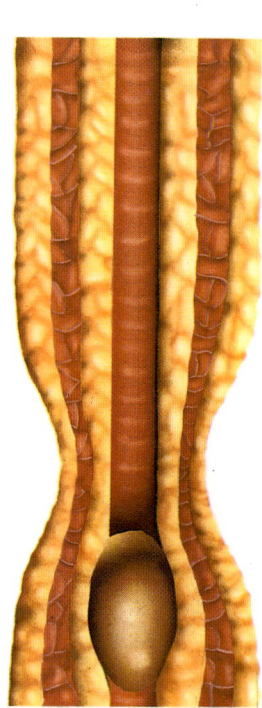

* Individual muscles are listed under muscles in the index and appear in *italics* in the text although they do not have glossary entries.

MOVING PARTS

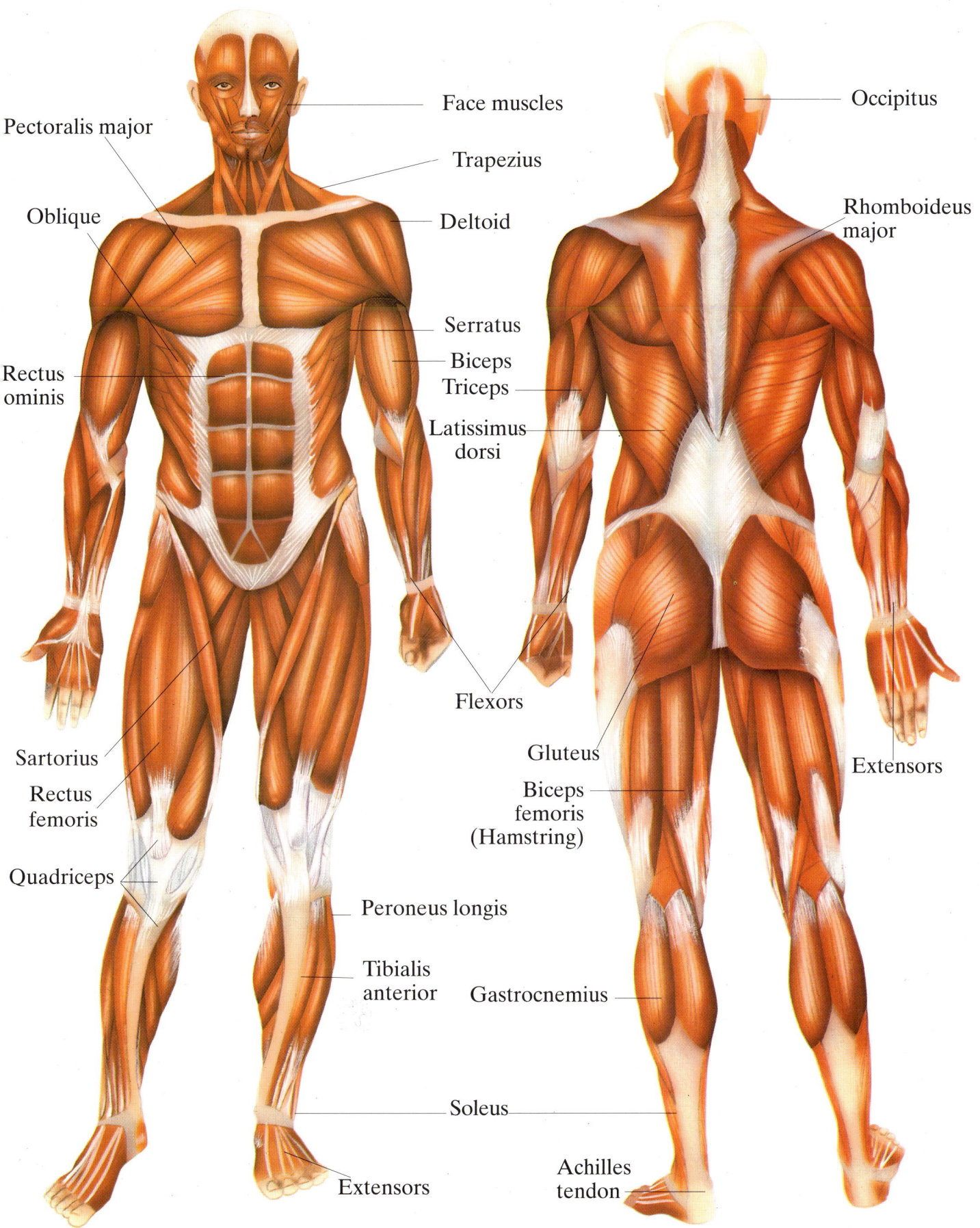

5

What are muscles made of?

There are three kinds of muscle tissue: voluntary, involuntary and cardiac. The voluntary muscles are also called skeletal muscles because they are attached to the bones of the skeleton. When you look at them under a microscope they appear striated or striped, which gives them the alternative name striated muscle.

These muscles are made up of long cells called muscle fibres. Each muscle cell has several nuclei. They also contain a number of thick *filaments* (threads) made of the protein *myosin*, and a number of thin filaments made of the protein *actin*. These filaments overlap one another and are arranged in regular patterns that show up as dark and light bands when you look at them under a microscope. The cells also contain mitochondria, where *oxygen* and *glucose* are 'burned' to make energy.

Each muscle fibre (cell) is wrapped in a very thin *membrane* or *sarcolemma*. Bundles of muscle cells are wrapped together in another membrane. These bundles also contain blood vessels which supply oxygen and *nutrients* to the muscles. Nerves which carry messages from the brain run to each cell.

Our muscles are made up of these bundles of muscle cells. The tiny muscles which move our eyelids contain only three bundles, wrapped in an outer membrane. Larger muscles contain many hundreds of bundles, again wrapped together in a smooth outer membrane that allows them to move easily past other surfaces.

Some muscles, such as those in the chest (*thorax*) and *abdomen* which help in breathing and protect our internal organs, are wide and flat. Long, spindle-shaped muscles move the bones of our arms and legs.

Our involuntary or smooth muscle tissue is made up of rather different cells. They are shaped like spindles, and each contains only one nucleus. These cells also contain many myosin and actin filaments, but they are not lined up regularly as in the voluntary muscles. The cells of smooth muscle tissue are arranged in flat sheets, and are found in the walls of organs with cavities, such as the stomach, and tubes such as blood vessels. Their contractions push along the contents, for example moving food through the *intestines*. Rings of muscle called *sphincters* act as 'gates', opening and closing to allow material through.

Cardiac muscle is made of branched cells with one or two nuclei. Its fibres are arranged in an orderly, criss-cross pattern.

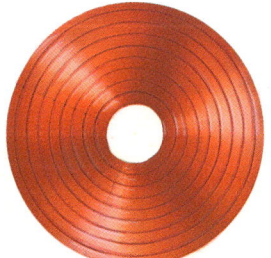

Circular

There are three different types of muscle tissue. Voluntary muscles are made of striated (striped) fibres. They are the muscles through which we control our movements. Cardiac muscle, found only in the heart, is also striped but the cells are differently shaped. Involuntary muscles are made up of smooth fibres. They line organs such as the stomach, intestines and blood vessels and we have no conscious control over them.

Muscles come in many different shapes – ring-shaped ones which close tubes in the body, short ones which help hold bones in place, wide, flat ones as in the abdomen, and bulging, spindle-shaped muscles as in the arms and legs.

Short

WHAT ARE MUSCLES MADE OF?

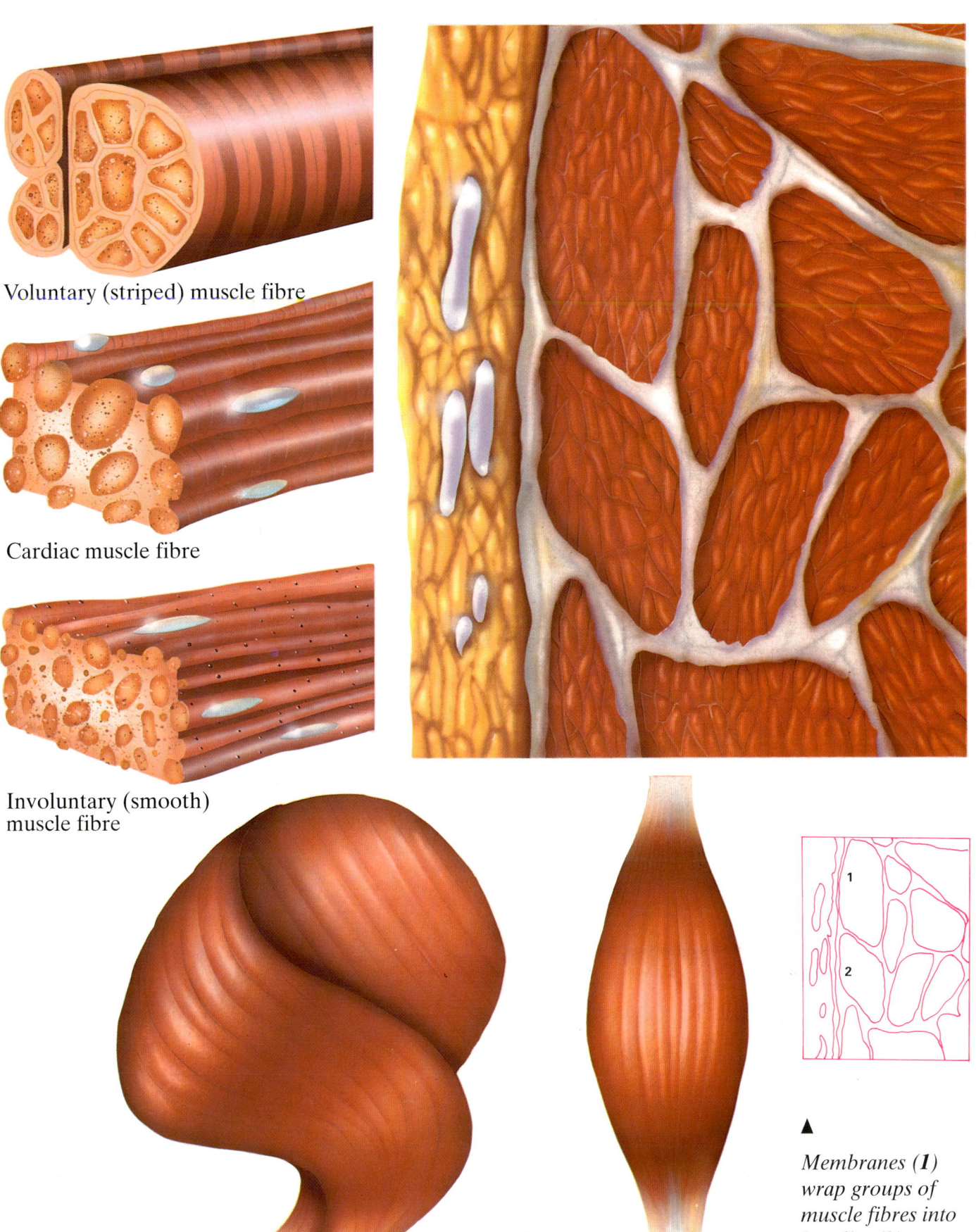

Voluntary (striped) muscle fibre

Cardiac muscle fibre

Involuntary (smooth) muscle fibre

Flat

Long

▲
Membranes (**1**) wrap groups of muscle fibres into bundles (**2**).

Into action

As we have seen, we have two main types of muscle tissue – voluntary and involuntary. The voluntary muscles are those which go to work when we want to move, and which hold our bones and organs in position.

Voluntary muscles are attached at either end, usually to two different bones but sometimes, as in the face, to skin or other soft tissue. Large muscles are attached to bones with tough connective tissue called *tendons*. Muscles make movements by contracting or shortening, sometimes by as much as 50 per cent, in response to nerve signals. They cannot relax and lengthen on their own; they need to be pulled back to their original shape by the action of other muscles.

One end of the muscle, called the origin, is attached to a bone which does not move. The other end, the insertion, is attached (often across a joint) to a bone which is moved when the muscle contracts.

Muscles often work in pairs, with a flexor muscle which bends a joint and an extensor muscle which straightens it again. For example, when the biceps muscle in the front of the upper arm contracts, the lower part of the arm bends upwards. To straighten the arm again, the triceps muscle at the back of the upper arm contracts. As it pulls the arm straight, the biceps relaxes and gets longer again.

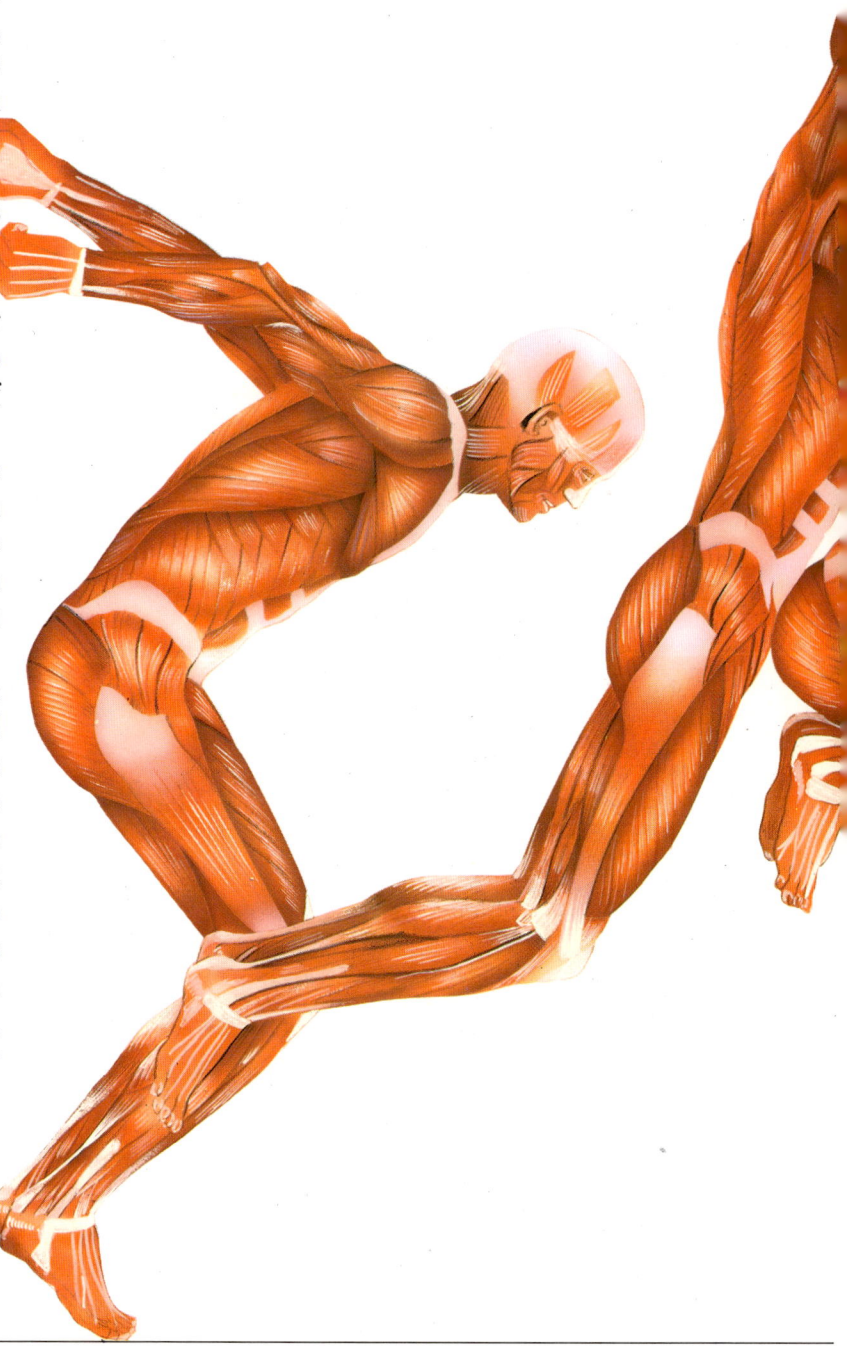

When you decide to jump, your brain sends signals to all the voluntary muscles involved in the action. Luckily you do not have to think of each individual message. ▼

INTO ACTION

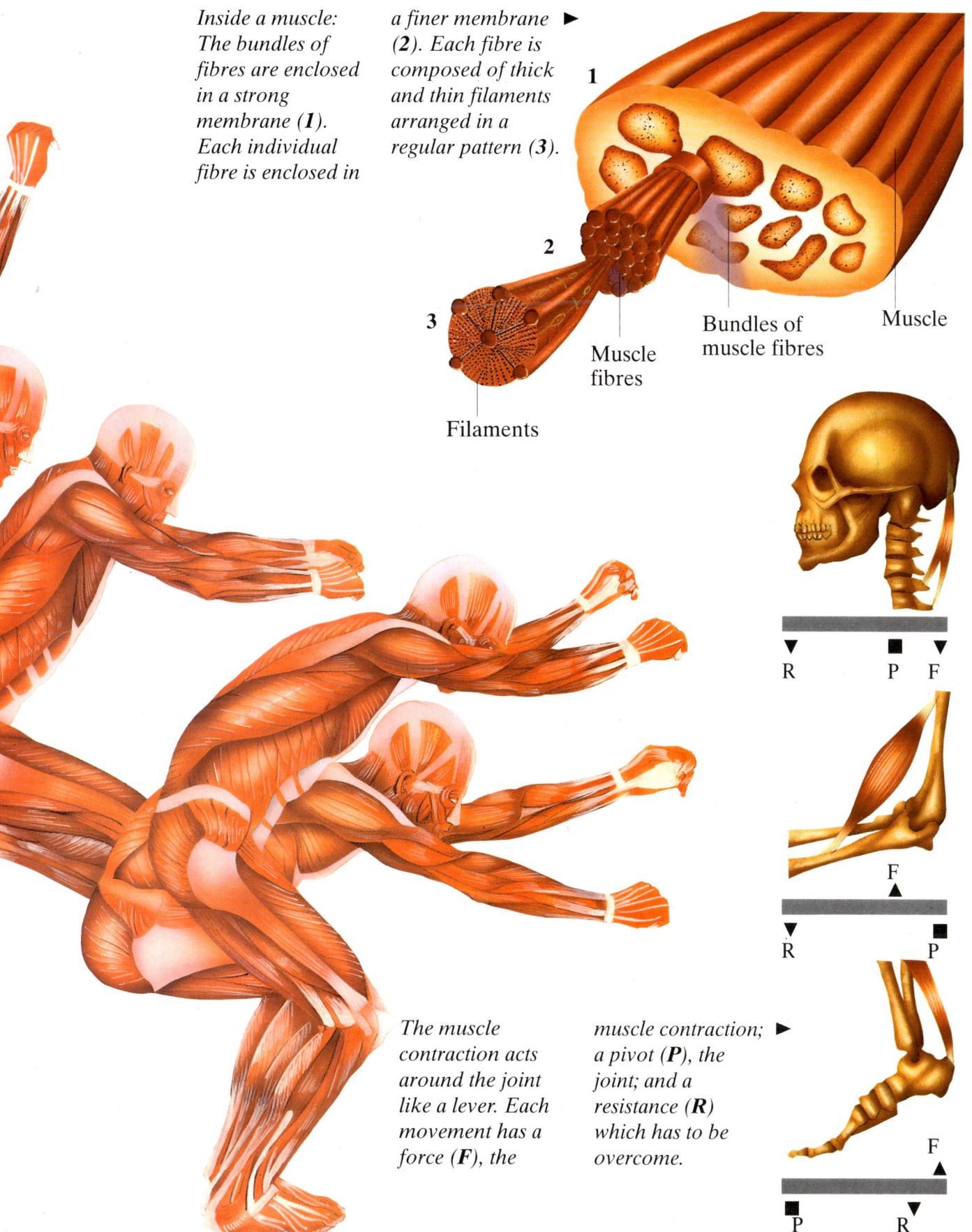

Inside a muscle: The bundles of fibres are enclosed in a strong membrane (**1**). Each individual fibre is enclosed in a finer membrane (**2**). Each fibre is composed of thick and thin filaments arranged in a regular pattern (**3**).

Filaments · Muscle fibres · Bundles of muscle fibres · Muscle

The muscle contraction acts around the joint like a lever. Each movement has a force (**F**), the muscle contraction; a pivot (**P**), the joint; and a resistance (**R**) which has to be overcome.

Energy factories

Muscles need energy for work. They get this from oxygen and glucose brought by the blood supply. This is called *aerobic metabolism*. When muscles are working gently, the ordinary flow of blood to the cell supplies enough oxygen and glucose for its needs. When you exercise, your muscles use up energy more rapidly; you breathe more quickly and deeply and your heart beats more strongly, to send an increased supply of oxygen and glucose to the muscles. When muscles are working and using up energy, they produce heat, so you feel warm.

Strenuous exercise can mean that the supply of oxygen runs out. The muscles then work in a different way. They use *anaerobic* (oxygenless) *metabolism* to release the energy from glucose, and they get much of the glucose from their own cells, where it is stored in a form called *glycogen*. But this form of metabolism is inefficient and cannot go on for long.

Aerobic metabolism produces the waste products *carbon dioxide* and water, which are carried away in the blood. Anaerobic metabolism produces the waste product *lactic acid*. This builds up in overworked muscles and makes them feel sore.

The number of muscle cells in the body always stays the same, but regular exercise can increase the size of each cell and so the muscles grow larger and stronger. Regular exercise also makes the body more efficient at supplying oxygen and glucose to the muscles – the *lungs* grow larger and the heart beats more strongly. When muscles are not used, they grow smaller and weaker.

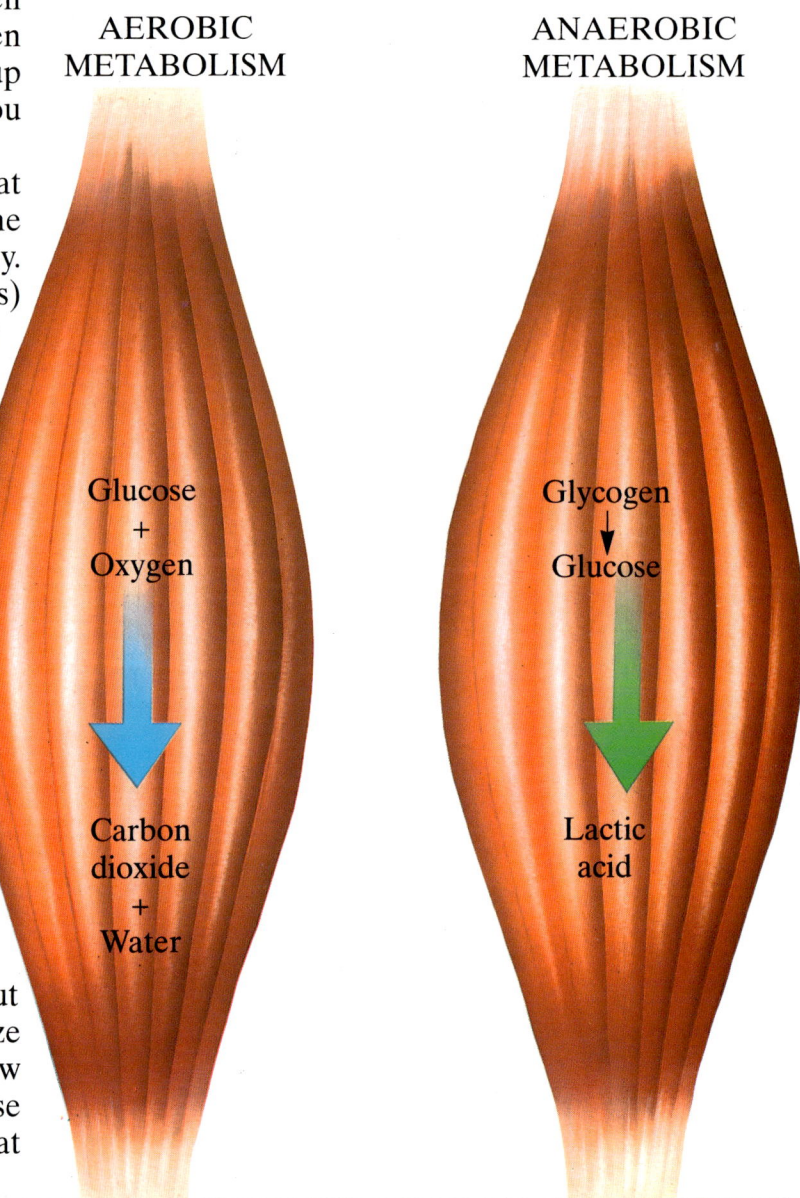

AEROBIC METABOLISM

Glucose + Oxygen

Carbon dioxide + Water

ANAEROBIC METABOLISM

Glycogen → Glucose

Lactic acid

ENERGY FACTORIES

When we exercise regularly and not too strenuously, the blood supplies our muscles with enough oxygen and glucose to provide the necessary energy. This produces the waste products carbon dioxide and water, in a process called aerobic metabolism. But if we do hard work without specially training for it, our muscles cannot get enough of their usual fuel. They get energy less efficiently by converting their stored glycogen into glucose and 'burning' it without oxygen in anaerobic metabolism. This forms lactic acid as a waste product, which causes stiffness.

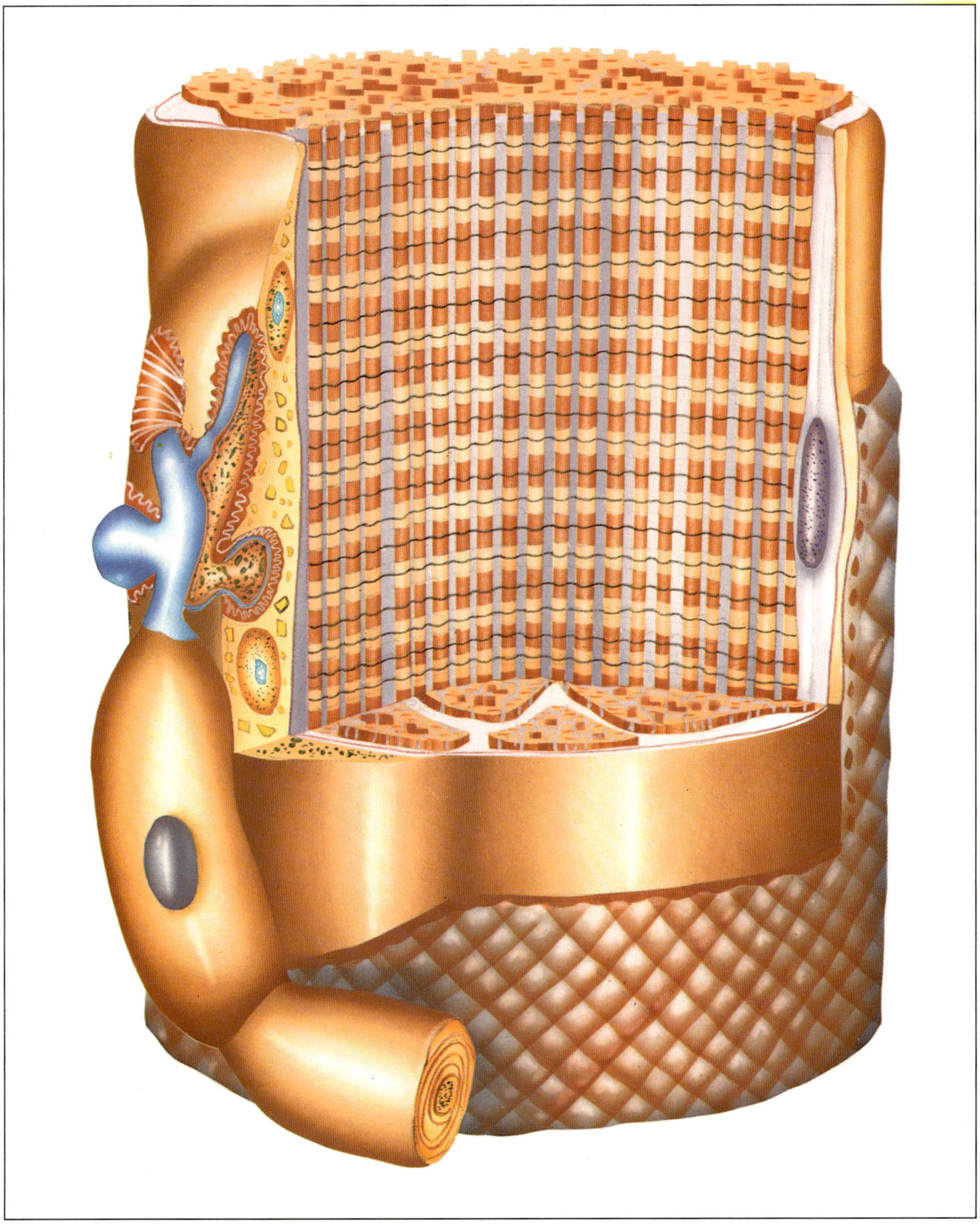

Muscle tissue is formed of bundles containing many long cells. Within these cells are protein filaments (**1**). There are thick filaments made of the protein myosin and thin filaments of the protein actin. In voluntary muscle tissue these are arranged in a regular pattern which produces a striped appearance (**2**). The filaments slide over one another during contraction.

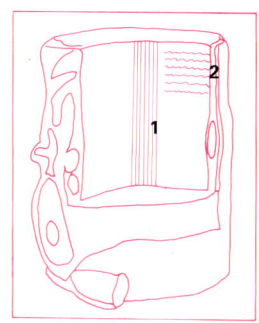

THE MUSCLES

Muscles, bones and joints

The bones of the skeleton – the body's framework – are supported and moved by muscles. These are attached at each end to bone or other tissue. Many muscles are attached on either side of joints – places where the bones of the skeleton are connected. Joints include the shoulder, elbow, wrist, hip, knee, ankle and neck.

The range of movements in a joint depends on the arrangement of the muscles around it and on the shape of the joint itself. The arm meets the shoulder in a ball and socket joint which allows movement in several directions – up and down, side to side, and rotation in a circle. The joint between the spine and the skull allows you to swivel your head around, but the hinge joint in your knee allows movement in one direction only.

Where two bones meet at a joint, their ends are covered with a layer of a smooth and flexible substance called *cartilage*. Over this is a smooth membrane which allows the bones to slide easily around. The joint is held in place by bands of strong, stretchy tissue called *ligaments*. The muscles have smooth outer membranes which let them slide easily past the bones and other tissues.

Muscles which move joints are attached to two bones. The origin of the muscle is the point of attachment nearest the centre of the body. The attachment at the other end is called the insertion. When a muscle contracts, the bone to which it is attached is pulled towards the bone of the origin, and the joint allows it to move smoothly into its new position.

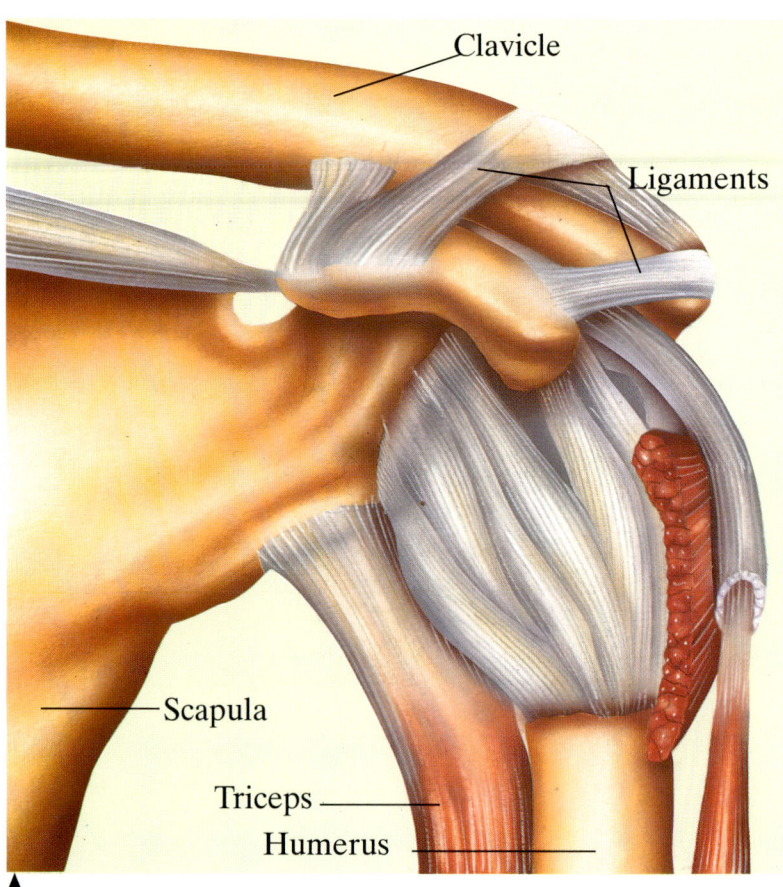

The shoulder can move in many directions – forwards and backwards, up and down, sideways and twisting around. The bone of the upper arm, the humerus, *ends in a ball shape, which fits into a cup-shaped socket in the shoulder blade (the* scapula*). Along the top is the collar bone or clavicle.*

The knee is a hinge joint between the thigh bone or femur, *which has a rounded end, and the shin bone or* tibia, *the end of which is saucer shaped. There are two halfmoon-shaped pads of specially fibrous cartilage, the* menisci, *on either side of the knee. They help the smooth action of the joint. The tendon of the* quadriceps *runs over the front of the knee, and within it is a bone called the* kneecap *or* patella.

MUSCLES, BONES AND JOINTS

The lower part of the leg has a number of muscles which work together to move the toes and turn the foot. Muscles originating in the thigh bend the lower leg towards the thigh. The large, powerful gluteus muscles of the buttock move the upper leg ▼

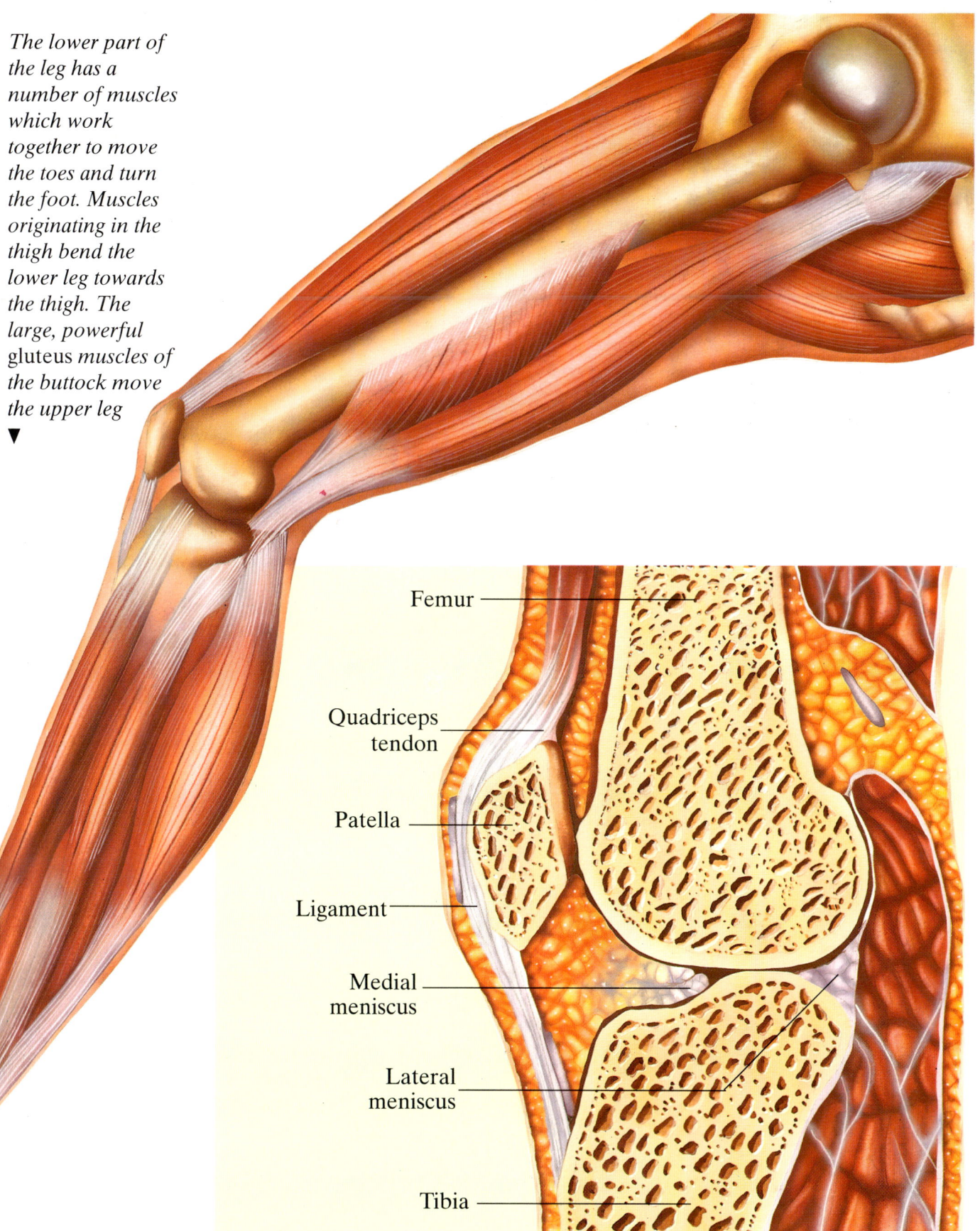

THE MUSCLES

Moving our limbs

The muscles of our arms and legs attach them to the trunk of the body and move them around. The top of the arm at the shoulder is covered by the thick and powerful *deltoid* muscle, which raises and turns it. The most important muscles of the upper arm are the *biceps* in the front, and the *triceps* at the back. These are 'antagonistic' muscles – they work as a pair to carry out opposing actions.

The forearm has muscles called *supinators* and *pronators*, which control the turning motion of the forearm and the rotation of the hands, and flexors and extensors which bend and straighten the fingers. The hand has small, short muscles which are purely for moving the fingers. The most important allow the thumb to touch the fingers in a pinch.

At the top of the leg are the *gluteus* muscles which form the buttocks. They keep the trunk of the body upright and balanced, and move the hip joint. On the front of the thigh is the powerful *quadriceps*, composed of the *rectus femoris, vastus medialis, vastus lateralis* and *vastus intermedius* muscles. They join together in the quadriceps tendon which runs over the knee. They flex the hip and extend and support the knee. On the inner side of the thigh are *adductor* muscles which raise the thigh and support the hip. On the back of the thigh is a group of muscles, including the *biceps femoris*, sometimes called the hamstring. It extends the hip and flexes the knee.

The major calf muscles are the *gastrocnemius* and the *soleus* muscles which flex and extend the foot while walking. They are attached to the bone of the heel by the Achilles tendon. The foot itself contains small muscles which move the toes and make it easier to walk.

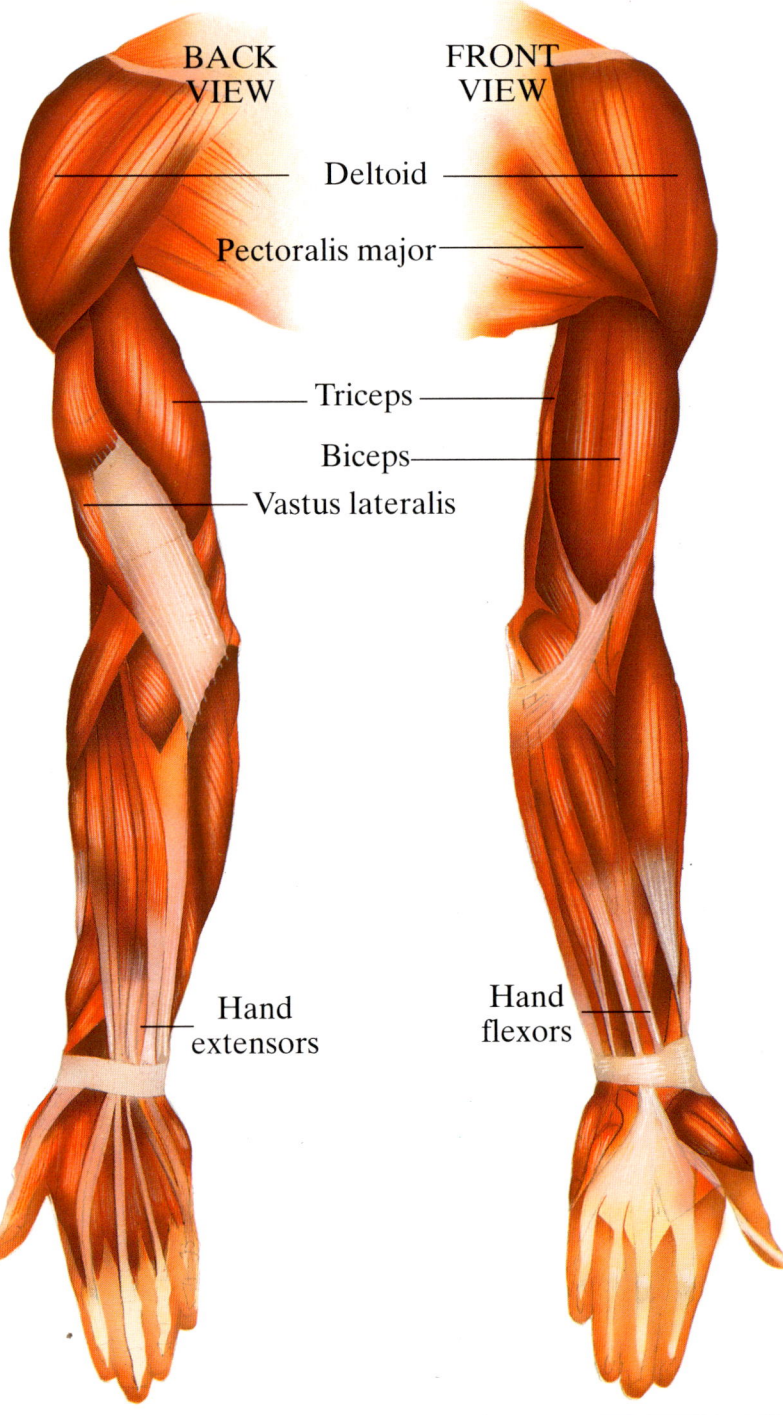

MOVING OUR LIMBS

The muscles at the front of the arm are mostly flexors, and those at the back extensors. The *deltoid* muscle links the arm to the shoulder and raises and turns it. In the front of the *arm is the* biceps, *which* draws up the lower arm; at the back is the triceps, *which* straightens it again. Other arm muscles turn the lower arms and move the hands.

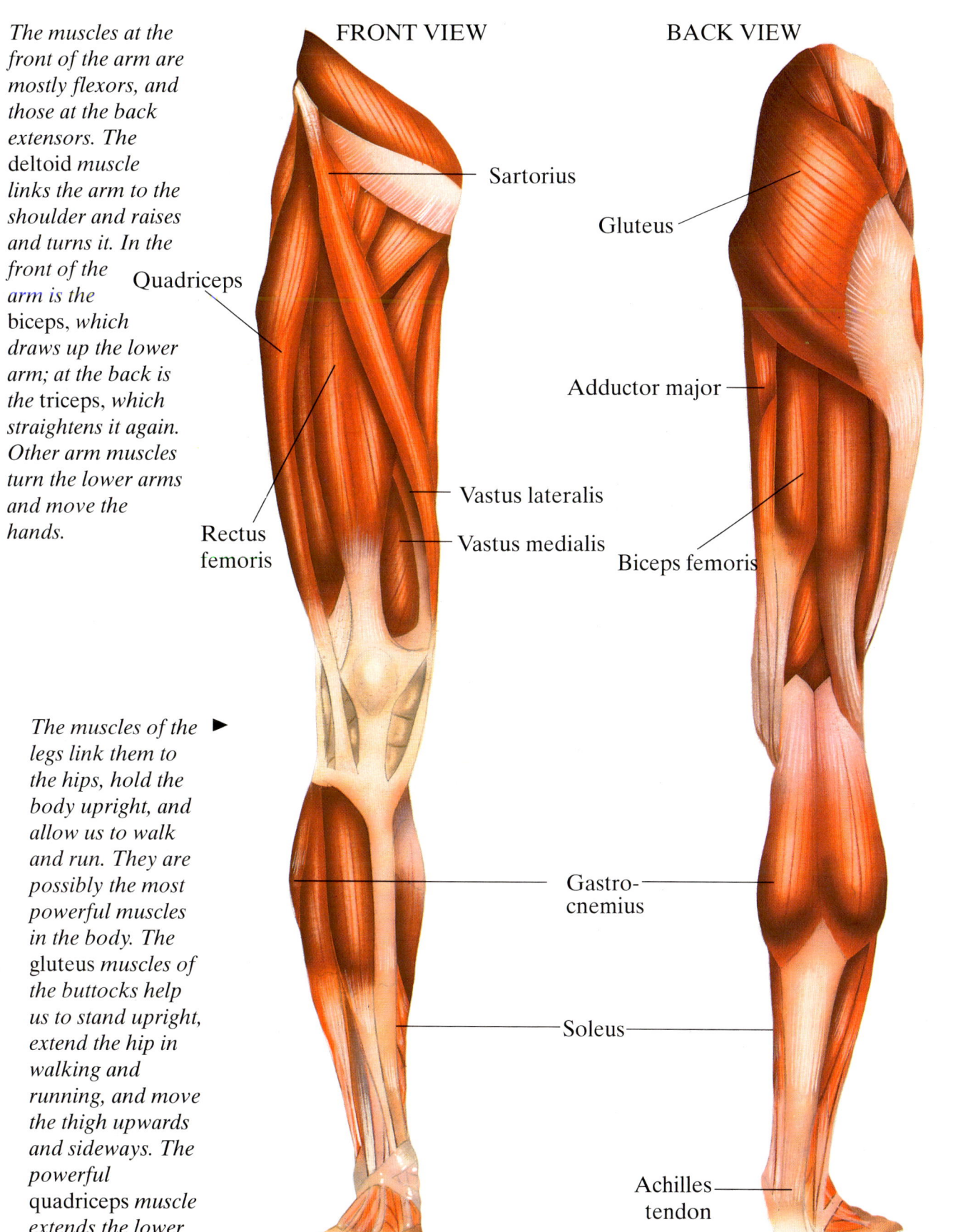

▶ The muscles of the legs link them to the hips, hold the body upright, and allow us to walk and run. They are possibly the most powerful muscles in the body. The gluteus *muscles of the buttocks help us to stand upright, extend the hip in walking and running, and move the thigh upwards and sideways. The powerful* quadriceps *muscle extends the lower leg.*

THE MUSCLES

Frowning, chewing and looking around

The muscles of the head and face vary from tiny muscles controlling delicate movements, such as those which move the eyeball, to the immensely powerful muscles of the jaw. They are divided into two groups. The facial muscles are mostly small, flat bands of muscle, attached at one end to bone or cartilage and at the other to skin. We use them to open, close and move our eyes, to move our lips, to sniff, and to show our feelings by smiling and frowning. The muscles of mastication (chewing), in contrast, are very powerful. They open and close the lower jaw and move it from side to side. We use these masseter and temporalis muscles when we clench our teeth. They are so strong that acrobats can support their whole body weight from a bar held between their teeth! People sometimes unconsciously clench their teeth when they are stressed, and this can give them bad jaw- and headaches.

The neck muscles control the movements of the head and hold it in position. The head is very heavy and needs strong muscles to keep it steady – a small baby's head rolls about alarmingly and needs supporting because its neck muscles are not yet strong enough to do the job. The sternomastoid muscle runs from behind the ear to the shoulder, and bends and swivels the head. The back of the neck is covered by the trapezius, a flat muscle which runs from the back of the skull down to the shoulder. Its function is to brace the shoulder and control movements of the shoulder and upper arm.

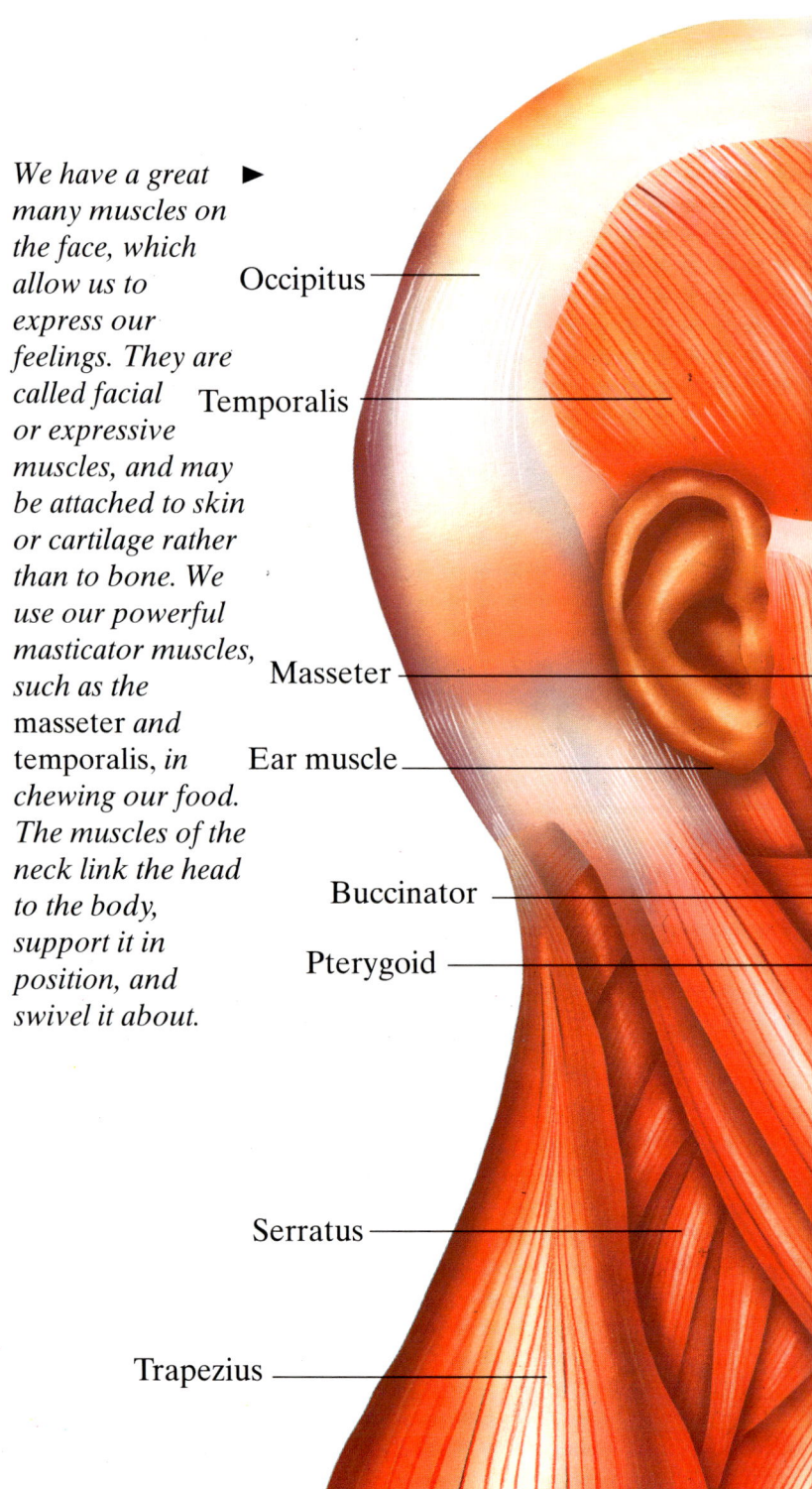

We have a great many muscles on the face, which allow us to express our feelings. They are called facial or expressive muscles, and may be attached to skin or cartilage rather than to bone. We use our powerful masticator muscles, such as the masseter *and* temporalis, *in chewing our food. The muscles of the neck link the head to the body, support it in position, and swivel it about.*

FROWNING, CHEWING AND LOOKING AROUND

The tiny muscles around the eye move the eyeball and the eyelid.

There are six voluntary muscles in the eye socket alone!

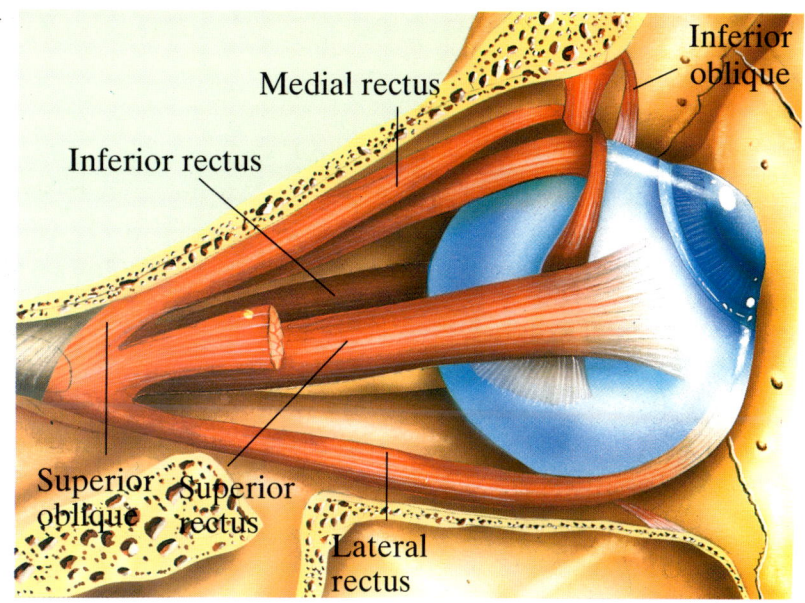

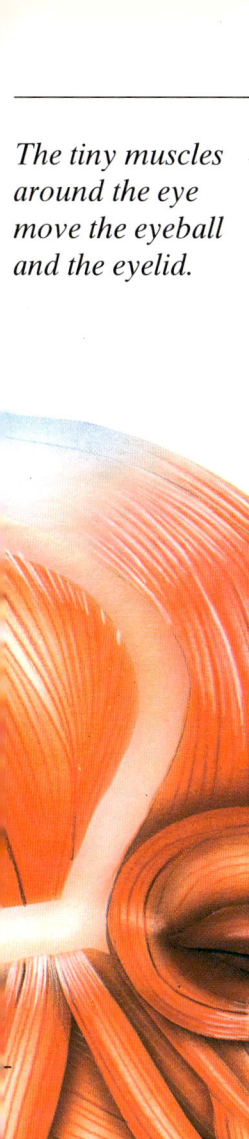

- Occipito frontalis
- Orbicularis oculi
- Zygomaticus
- Orbicularis oris
- Infrahyoid
- Sternomastoid

Some muscles of the face are attached to the skin. This is made up of the epidermis and dermis with a subcutaneous layer of fat beneath. The skin contains a network of fibres which give it great elasticity and resistance.

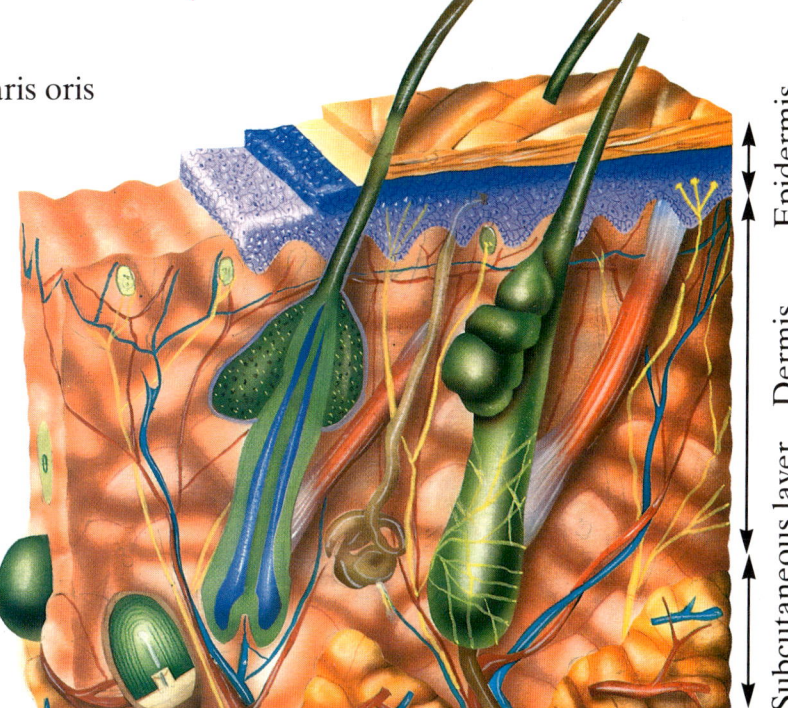

THE MUSCLES

In your trunk

The area of the body between the shoulders and the pelvis, known as the trunk, has two parts. The upper part is called the chest, or thorax. It contains vital organs including the heart and lungs, protected by the bones of the thoracic cage. The most obvious muscles on the chest, are involved in raising and rotating the arms. These muscles are the *pectorals* and the *serratus*. Below the chest is the abdomen, containing the stomach and the intestines. They are held in position by bracing flat sheets of muscle, which also control the bending of the body at the waist.

The chest and abdomen are separated by a dome-shaped sheet of muscle called the *diaphragm*. It is connected by muscle fibres to the lower ribs, the breastbone (*sternum*) and the spine, and plays a vital part in our breathing. At rest, the diaphragm curves up into the chest (thoracic) cavity in a dome. When we breathe in, the muscles of the diaphragm contract and it flattens into the abdomen. This enlarges the space in the chest cavity, the lungs expand, and air is drawn into them. When the diaphragm relaxes again, it rises back into the chest, the lungs have less room and air is driven out of them. This happens about 20 times a minute without our thinking about it, but we can deliberately change the speed of breathing by panting or holding the breath. Sometimes the diaphragm contracts and relaxes in spasms which we cannot control. The result is painful *hiccups*.

Other muscles used in breathing are the *intercostals*. These move the ribs outwards and upwards, enlarging the chest cavity.

The abdominal cavity is completely surrounded by muscles which protect its contents and keep them in place. The most important muscles are the rectus abdominis, *which runs between the breastbone and the pelvis, and the oblique* muscles on the side of the abdomen.

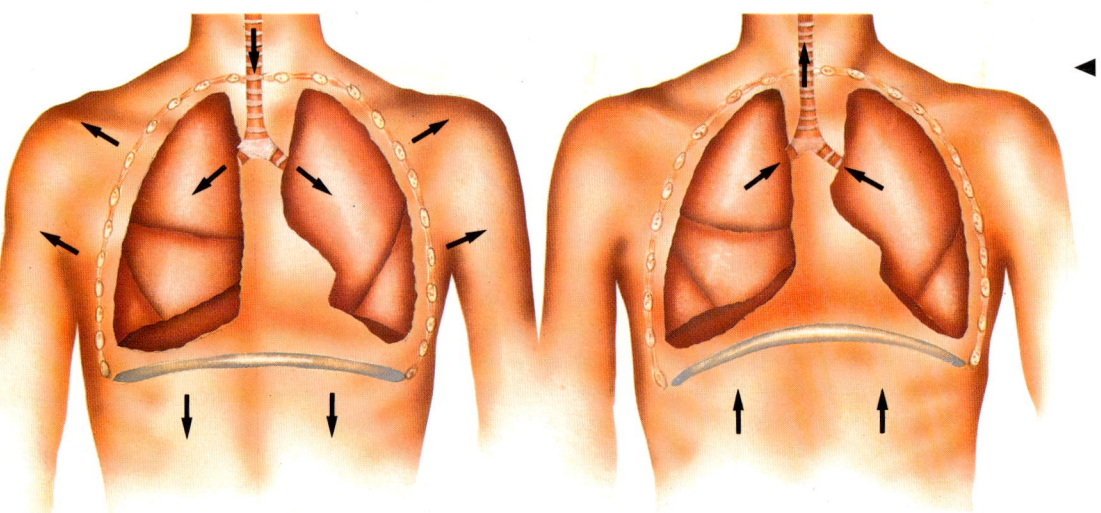

Breathing in　　　　　Breathing out

◀ *When we inhale, the diaphragm flattens downwards, increasing the size of the chest cavity. When we breathe out, the diaphragm relaxes and rises into the cavity.*

IN YOUR TRUNK

Some of the muscles at the top of the chest are joined at one end to the chest and at the other to the upper arm. These include the deltoid, pectoral *and* serratus *muscles, the function of which is to move the shoulder and arm. Other chest muscles which lie in a deeper layer include the* intercostal *muscles, that move the ribs.*

▼

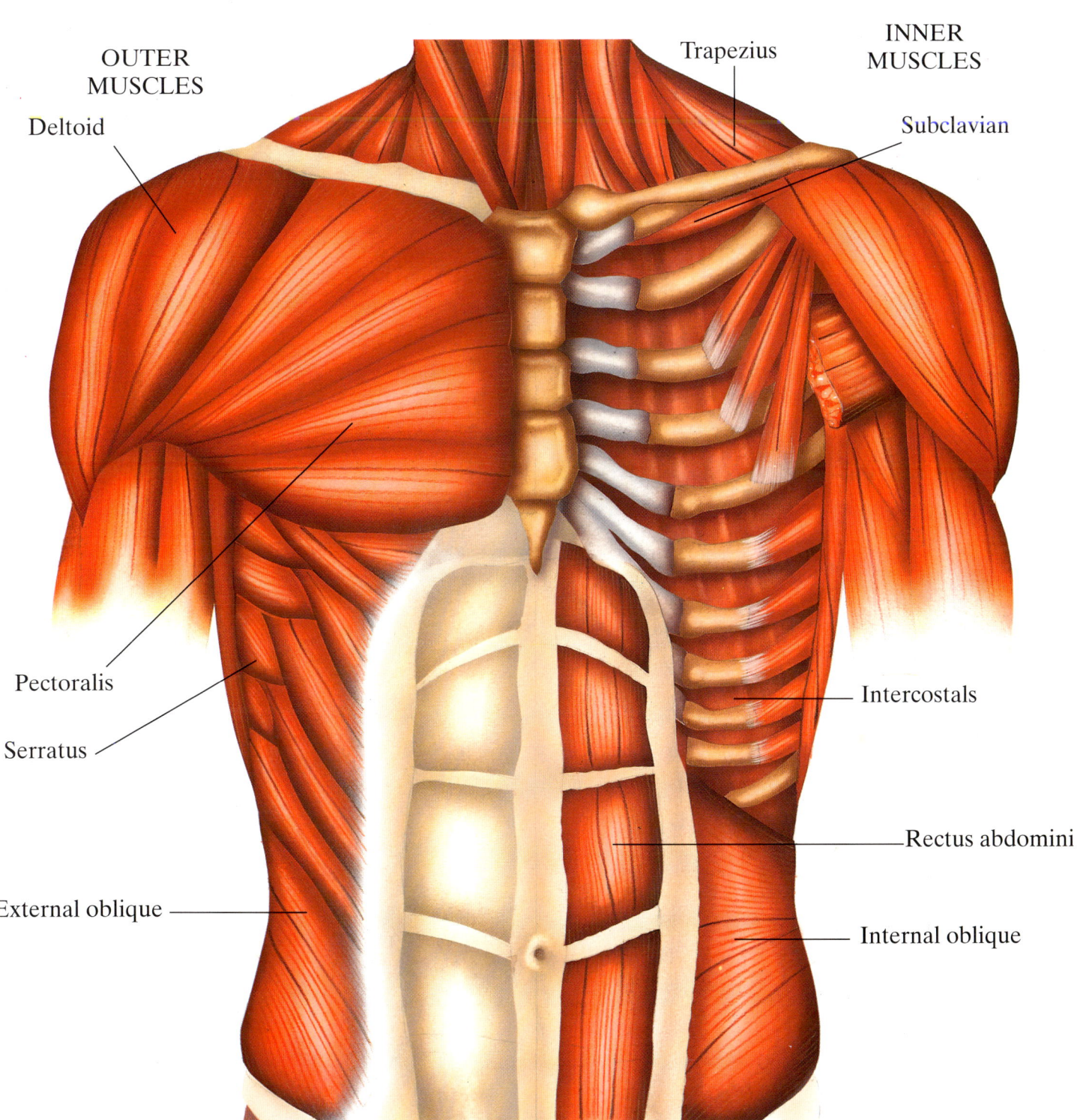

OUTER MUSCLES
- Deltoid
- Pectoralis
- Serratus
- External oblique

Trapezius

INNER MUSCLES
- Subclavian
- Intercostals
- Rectus abdomini
- Internal oblique

THE MUSCLES

Processing food

We use our muscles to eat and digest our food. This process starts in the mouth, when our powerful jaw muscles enable our teeth to crush and grind food into small pieces. These are voluntary muscles. The food then begins a long journey down the digestive tract, a series of tubes and cavities the walls of which contain rings and lengthwise bands of involuntary (smooth) muscle. This acts without our conscious control. The food is moved along the digestive tract by rhythmic contractions known as peristaltic waves. All along the tract, muscles contract behind the food and relax in front of it, pushing it along on its journey. At the same time, they pummel it into smaller and smaller pieces.

A ball, or *bolus*, of chewed food mixed with saliva is directed by the tongue, a thick bundle of membrane-covered muscle, through the back of the mouth into the oesophagus. This is a tube about 25 centimetres long which leads down to the stomach. Here the food is mixed with digestive juices which help to break it down into small fragments. Strong contractions of the stomach's muscular walls churn the mixture into a creamy substance called *chyme*. At the far end of the stomach is a ring of muscle called the pyloric sphincter. It relaxes to allow small amounts of chyme through to the intestines. As the food moves through them, still propelled by peristaltic waves, nutrients pass from it into the blood and are carried round the body. The unusable waste passes into the rectum and is expelled from the body through the *anus*, which is normally closed by two rings of muscle or sphincters.

The smooth muscles are controlled automatically by nerves over which we have no conscious control, and by hormones. These can be affected by stress, so when you are nervous or upset you may find that you do not feel like eating.

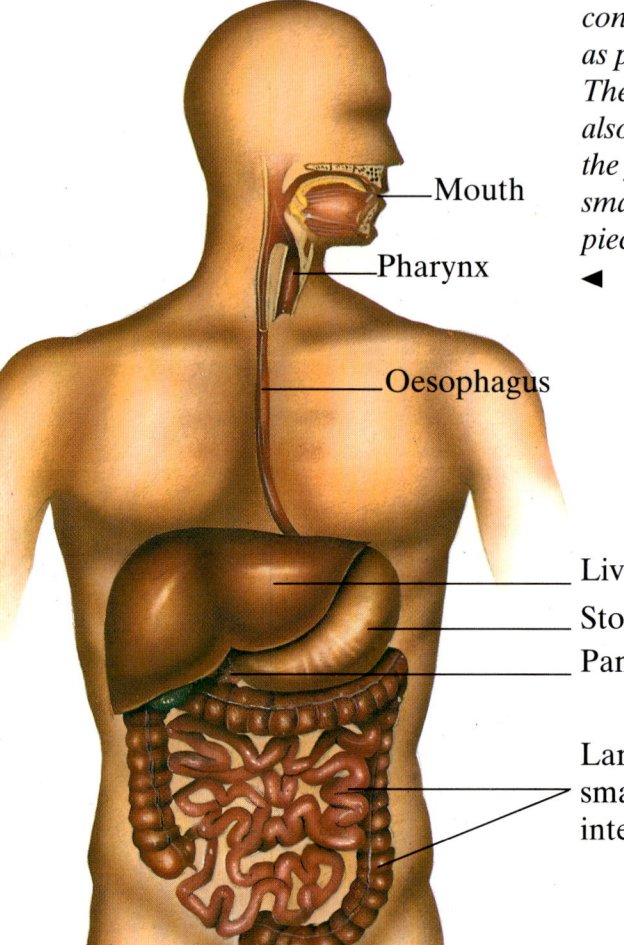

The digestive tract is a long tube which runs from the mouth through the stomach to the anus and is between 10 and 12 metres long. The walls of the digestive tract are lined with involuntary (smooth) muscle that propels the food along by a series of muscular contractions known as peristaltic waves. These movements also help to break the food down into smaller and smaller pieces. ◄

PROCESSING FOOD

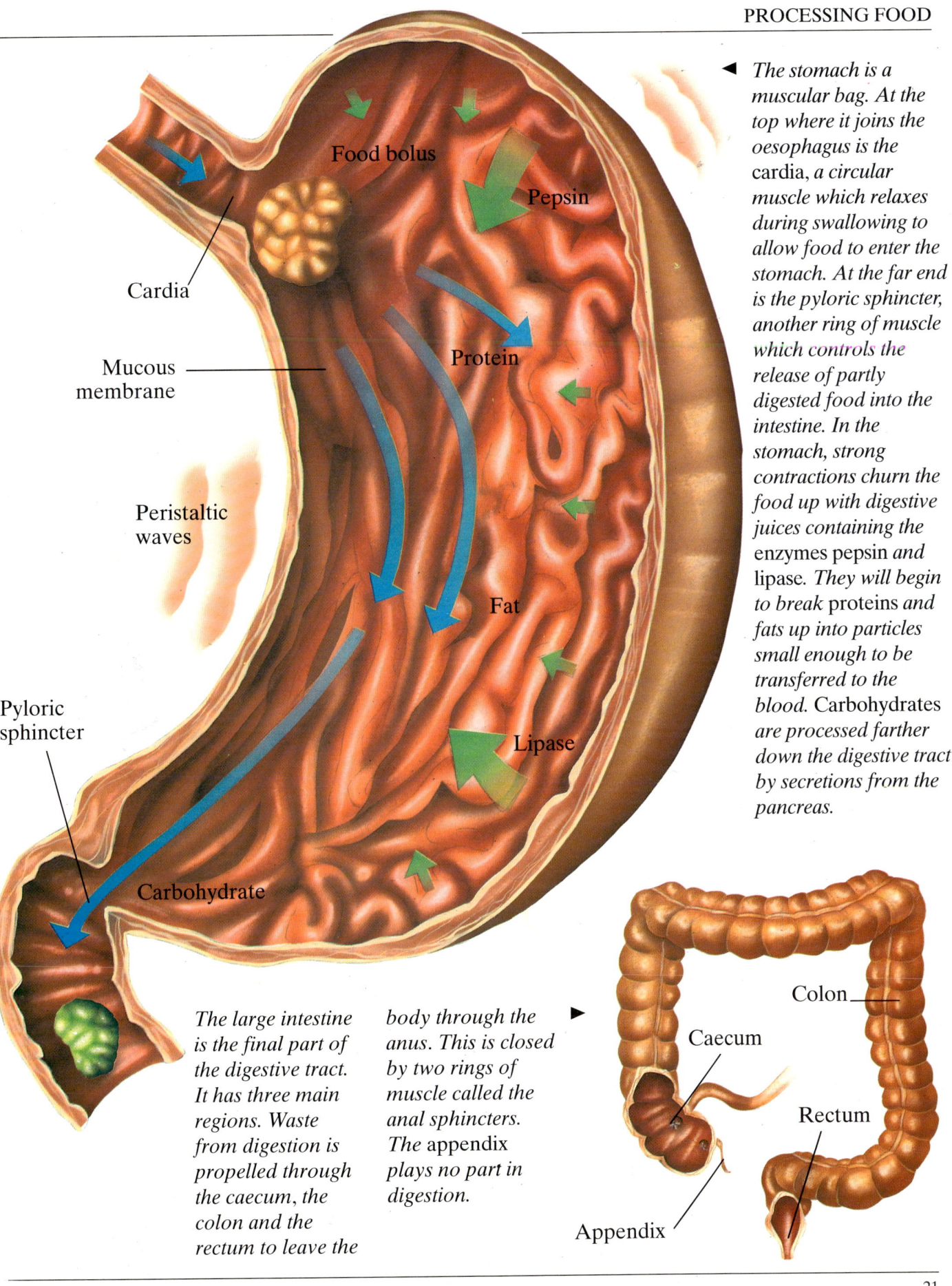

◀ The stomach is a muscular bag. At the top where it joins the oesophagus is the cardia, a circular muscle which relaxes during swallowing to allow food to enter the stomach. At the far end is the pyloric sphincter, another ring of muscle which controls the release of partly digested food into the intestine. In the stomach, strong contractions churn the food up with digestive juices containing the enzymes pepsin and lipase. They will begin to break proteins and fats up into particles small enough to be transferred to the blood. Carbohydrates are processed farther down the digestive tract by secretions from the pancreas.

▶ The large intestine is the final part of the digestive tract. It has three main regions. Waste from digestion is propelled through the caecum, the colon and the rectum to leave the body through the anus. This is closed by two rings of muscle called the anal sphincters. The appendix plays no part in digestion.

Moving the blood

The body's supply of oxygen and nutrients is carried round by the blood. This is pumped from the heart through a system of *arteries, arterioles, capillaries* and *veins* which reach every part of the body. As it flows round the body, the blood exchanges nutrients for waste products. It flows back to the heart and through the lungs where it picks up oxygen before returning to the heart and starting its journey again.

The heart itself is made of a special type of muscle called cardiac muscle. The arteries, arterioles (smaller arteries) and veins all have a layer of involuntary (smooth) muscle in their walls.

The muscular walls of the arterioles can control the flow of blood to an area of the body. Tissues need a good supply of blood when they are working and the arterioles let this through. They can close to shut off the tiny capillaries leading to areas at rest, directing the blood instead to small veins from which it will flow back to the heart. They also help regulate the body's temperature; when you are hot, your skin flushes as extra blood is directed to the body's surface where heat can be dispersed. The opposite happens when you are cold: the tiny blood vessels near the surface are shut off to conserve heat in the body.

As it circulates through the body, blood has to flow upwards, against gravity, on its way back to the heart. It needs an extra push to propel it on its way. The muscles in the veins are rather weak and cannot by themselves pump blood back to the heart, especially from the legs and abdomen. The upward movement of the blood is helped by movements of the surrounding muscles when we walk and move. The veins are squeezed, and valves in them ensure that the blood goes upwards and not back down.

These smooth muscles are usually not under our conscious control (though some people are able to train their bodies to respond to their will to some extent, for example by slowing down their heartbeat).

The body has twin circulatory systems. In the minor, or pulmonary, circulation, blood carrying the waste product carbon dioxide leaves the right side of heart through the pulmonary artery and is carried to the lungs, where it releases the carbon dioxide and absorbs oxygen. It then returns to the left side of the heart through the pulmonary veins.

▼

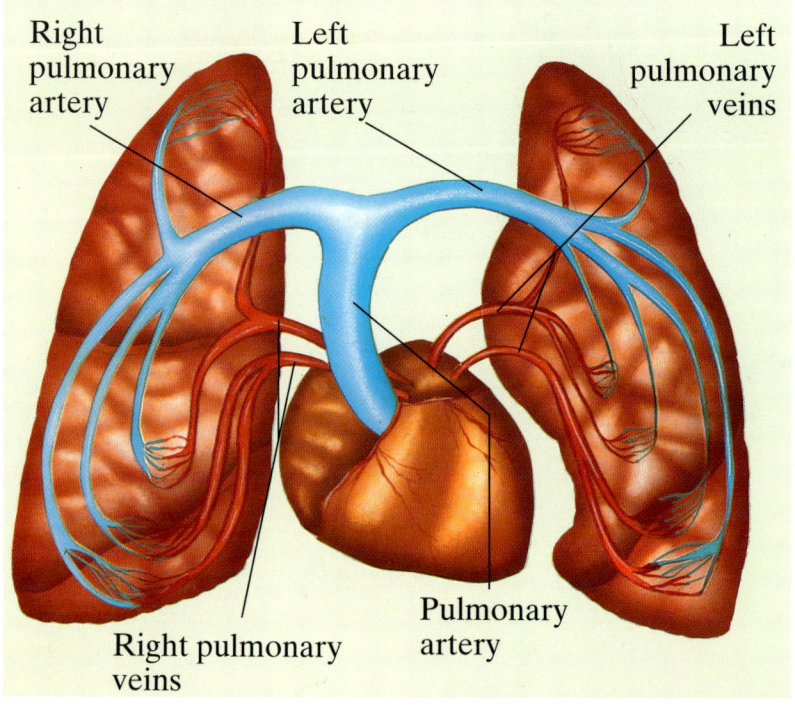

MOVING THE BLOOD

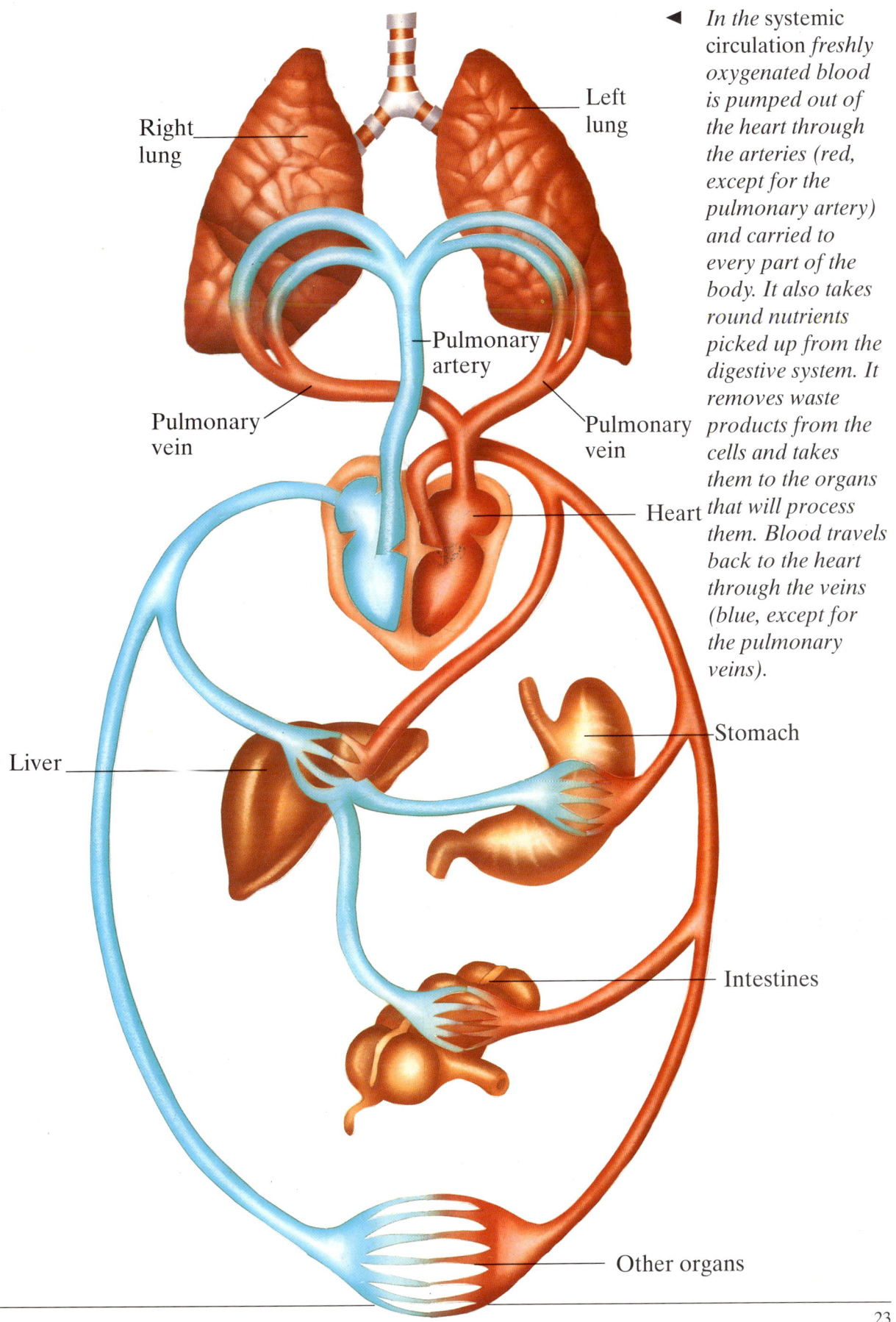

◀ *In the* systemic circulation *freshly oxygenated blood is pumped out of the heart through the arteries (red, except for the pulmonary artery) and carried to every part of the body. It also takes round nutrients picked up from the digestive system. It removes waste products from the cells and takes them to the organs that will process them. Blood travels back to the heart through the veins (blue, except for the pulmonary veins).*

The most important muscle

The most important organ in the body is the heart. It is a hollow organ, about the size of a fist, made of a special type of muscle called cardiac muscle. The cells of cardiac muscle are branched, and contain one or two nuclei. Like the cells of voluntary muscle, they contain thick and thin filaments, though these are not arranged in such an orderly pattern. This sort of muscle is found only in the heart. It is not a voluntary muscle – only a very few people ever learn how to control the rate of their heart beat. A normal heart beats about 70 times a minute – about 37 million times a year; and it goes on beating all through your life.

The heart lies in the chest and pumps blood around the body, through the circulatory system. Without it, we cannot live, since blood carries the oxygen and nutrients we need for our cells to work. During exercise, when the muscles need more oxygen, the heart beats faster to pump more blood round your body. When you are frightened your heart beat speeds up so that your muscles are ready for hard work if necessary; this is known as the 'fight or flight' reaction!

The heart has four sections called chambers. Blood from the veins, carrying the waste product carbon dioxide, flows into the upper right chamber or *atrium*. It is pumped into the lower right chamber or *ventricle* and then to the lungs, where the carbon dioxide is exchanged for oxygen. The freshly oxygenated blood flows from the lungs to the heart's left atrium, and is pumped through the left ventricle into the arteries which supply the body.

The muscle of the heart needs a good blood supply of its own to carry out its strenuous work; this is supplied by special coronary arteries.

Each side of the heart has two chambers. The upper chambers, the atria or auricles, have thin walls and dilate when blood enters them. They are connected by valves to two lower chambers called ventricles, which have larger, thicker walls. The left side of the heart is more muscular than the right; it pumps blood round the body, while the right side pumps it on a far shorter journey through the lungs.

A section of the special cardiac muscle which forms the heart. The arrangement of its fibres helps it to contract strongly and efficiently for many years.

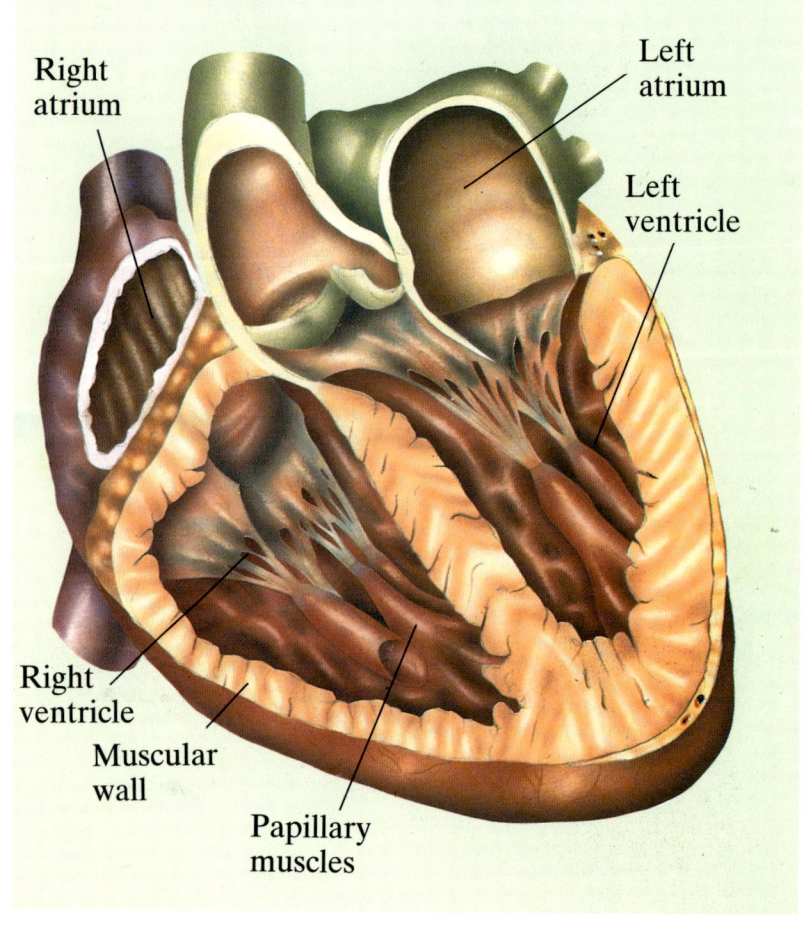

THE MOST IMPORTANT MUSCLE

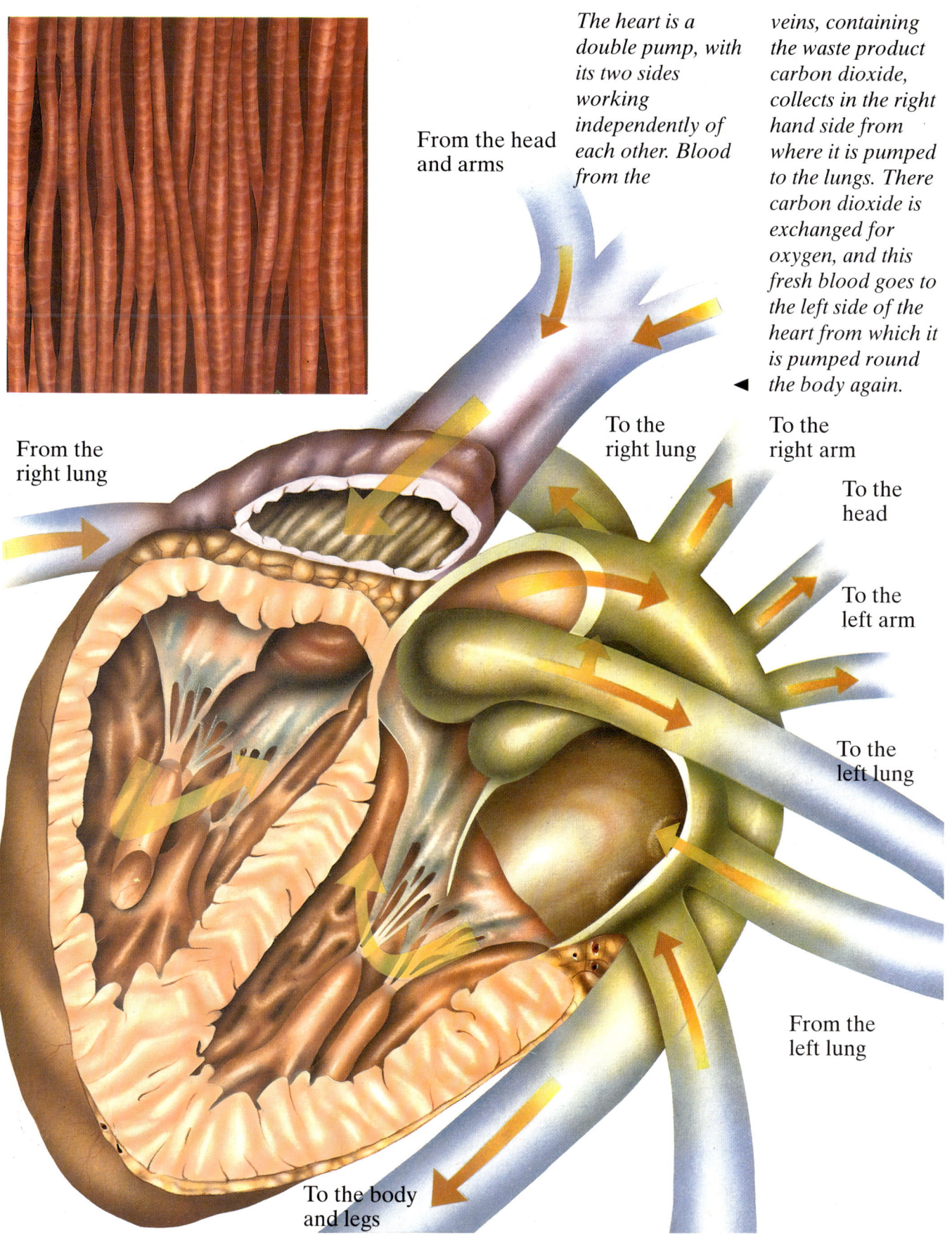

The heart is a double pump, with its two sides working independently of each other. Blood from the veins, containing the waste product carbon dioxide, collects in the right hand side from where it is pumped to the lungs. There carbon dioxide is exchanged for oxygen, and this fresh blood goes to the left side of the heart from which it is pumped round the body again.

From the head and arms

From the right lung

To the right lung

To the right arm

To the head

To the left arm

To the left lung

From the left lung

To the body and legs

25

Exercise and eat

Healthy muscles are strong and firm, and with their help our bodies function well. It is up to us to look after them. Muscles in good condition are less likely to be strained and torn. Muscles which are not used soon grow small and weak; anyone who has had an arm or leg in plaster for some time will know how feeble and wasted its muscles are when the plaster comes off. We cannot increase the number of fibres in a muscle, but we can make them larger and stronger by exercise.

Sensible exercise not only strengthens our muscles, but makes our heart and lungs more efficient too. When we exercise, the heart must send more blood to the muscles to provide them with enough oxygen and glucose, while the lungs need to draw in more oxygen for the blood. Athletes' hearts tend to beat more slowly than the average when they are at rest, because each beat is stronger and more efficient than in a less fit person.

Regular hard exercise is best. You should work hard enough to make you pant and increase your heartbeat, for about 20 minutes at a time. Always start with gentle exercises to warm the muscles up, otherwise you may strain them; and end with gentle exercises too. Running, walking and swimming are particularly good for you because they use most of the muscles in the body. Special weight training can strengthen particular muscles, but this does not improve general health.

Healthy eating helps build up healthy muscles. Make sure that you eat a sensible mixed diet, including carbohydrates, protein and fat, with plenty of fresh vegetables. They will provide you with all the nutrients that you need.

Our food should include body-building proteins, carbohydrates, and fats, which all produce energy; fibre, vitamins and minerals are also essential. And, of course, we cannot survive without water! A healthy diet includes fresh fruit and vegetables, cereals, milk, eggs, fish and meat; we should cut down on chocolate and other sweet things.

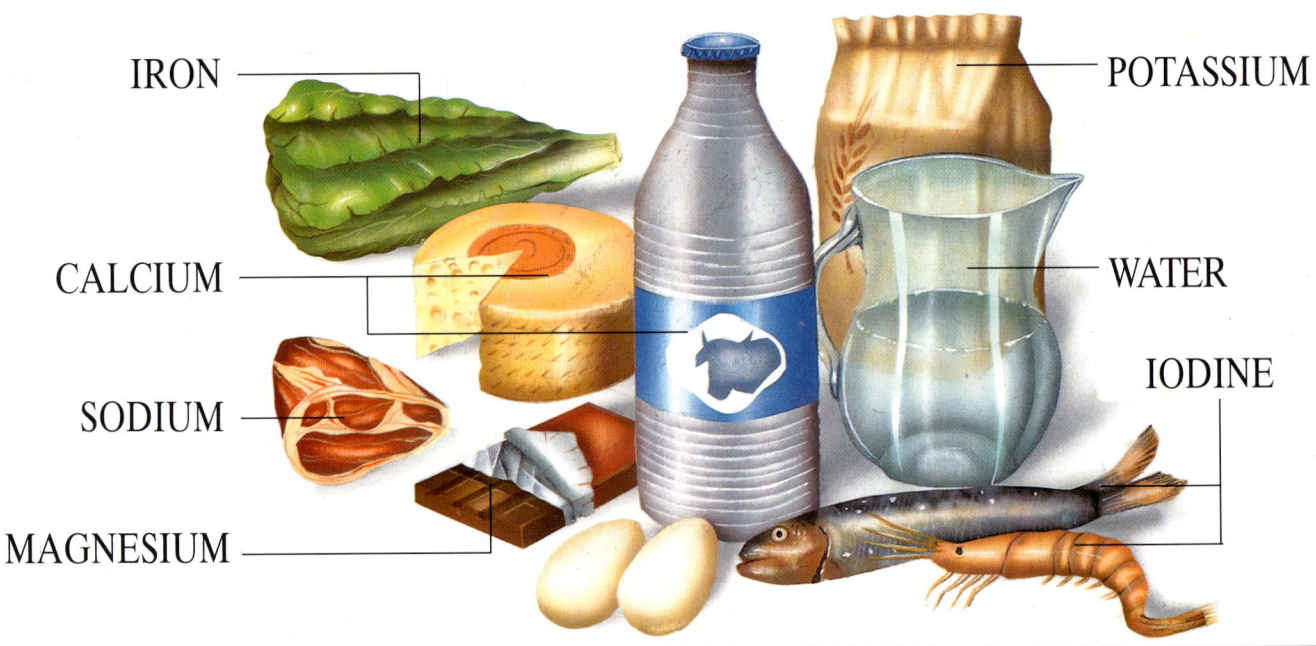

EXERCISE AND EAT

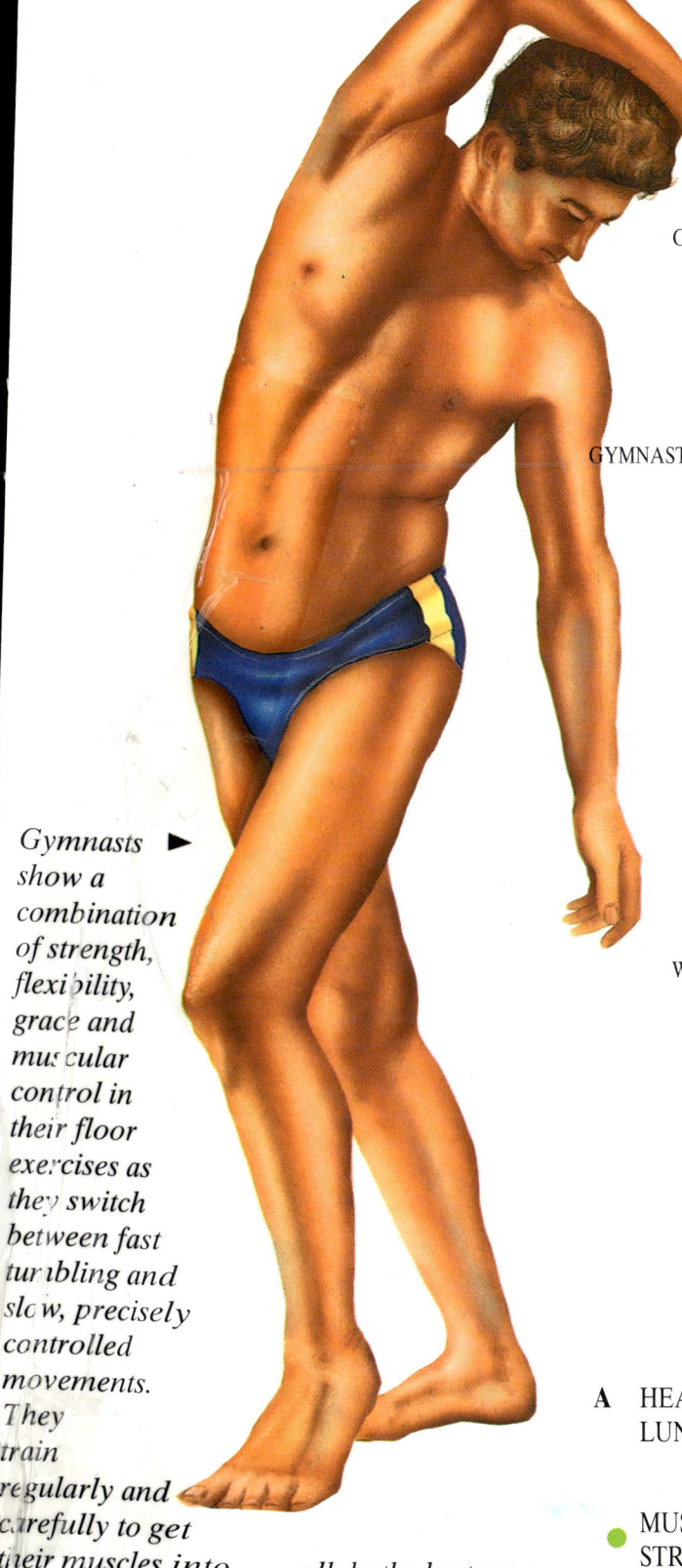

▶ Gymnasts show a combination of strength, flexibility, grace and muscular control in their floor exercises as they switch between fast tumbling and slow, precisely controlled movements. They train regularly and carefully to get their muscles into the best possible condition. Not all of us can do as well, but we should all do the best we can with our bodies by exercising regularly.

	BACK	SHOULDERS	ARMS	ABDOMEN	HIPS	LEGS	A
CROSS-COUNTRY RUNNING	🔴			🔴		🟢🔴🔵	⚫
SWIMMING	🟢🔴	🟢🔴🔵		🟢🔴	🔵	🟢🔵	⚫
BASKETBALL						🟢🔴🔵	⚫
WATER-SKIING	🔴		🟢🔴	🔴		🟢🔴	⚫
GYMNASTICS: vaulting horse	🟢		🟢🔵🔵	🟢	🔵		
vaulting beam	🟢		🔵	🟢		🟢🔵	
floor exercises	🟢	🔵	🟢🔴🟢		🔵	🟢🔵	
horizontal bar	🟢	🔵	🟢🔴🟢				
parallel bars	🟢	🔵	🟢			🔵	
rings	🟢	🔵	🟢🔴		🔵		
TENNIS		🔵				🟢🔴🔵	⚫
BOXING	🟢🔴	🟢🔴	🟢🔴	🟢🔴		🟢🔴	⚫
FENCING		🔵			🟢	🟢🔵	⚫
JUDO	🟢		🟢🔴🟢	🟢🔴	🔵	🟢🔴🔵	⚫
KARATE	🔴	🟢🔴	🟢🔴🟢	🟢🔴	🔵	🟢🔴🔴	⚫
WEIGHT-LIFTING	🟢🔴		🟢🔴			🟢🔴	
WRESTLING	🟢🔴	🔵	🟢🔴🔴	🟢🔴	🔵	🟢🔴🔵	⚫
BASEBALL		🔵		🔵		🔵	
HOCKEY	🔴		🔵			🟢🔴🔵	
ICE-HOCKEY	🟢		🟢	🟢	🔵	🟢	⚫
RUGBY			🟢			🟢🔴🔵	⚫
FOOTBALL						🟢🔴🔵	⚫
WATER-POLO	🔴	🔵	🟢🔴			🔴	⚫

A — HEART AND LUNG FITNESS

🟢 MUSCLE STRENGTH

🔴 ENDURANCE

🔵 FLEXIBILITY

▲ Different kinds of sport and exercise help our fitness in different ways. This table shows how some common activities affect our bodies when they are carried out properly

THE MUSCLES

Finding out

The more we find out about our muscles, the more fascinating – and sometimes strange – things we learn about the way in which they control our bodies.

Fast-moving muscles
One of the fastest-moving voluntary muscles of the body is the one that opens and shuts the eyelids. We can blink up to five times a second – try it! This is very slow indeed compared to the muscle movements made by some other animals. Some hummingbirds beat their wings about 80 times a second, and some species of insects can beat their wings a thousand times a second – the fastest muscle movement we know of.

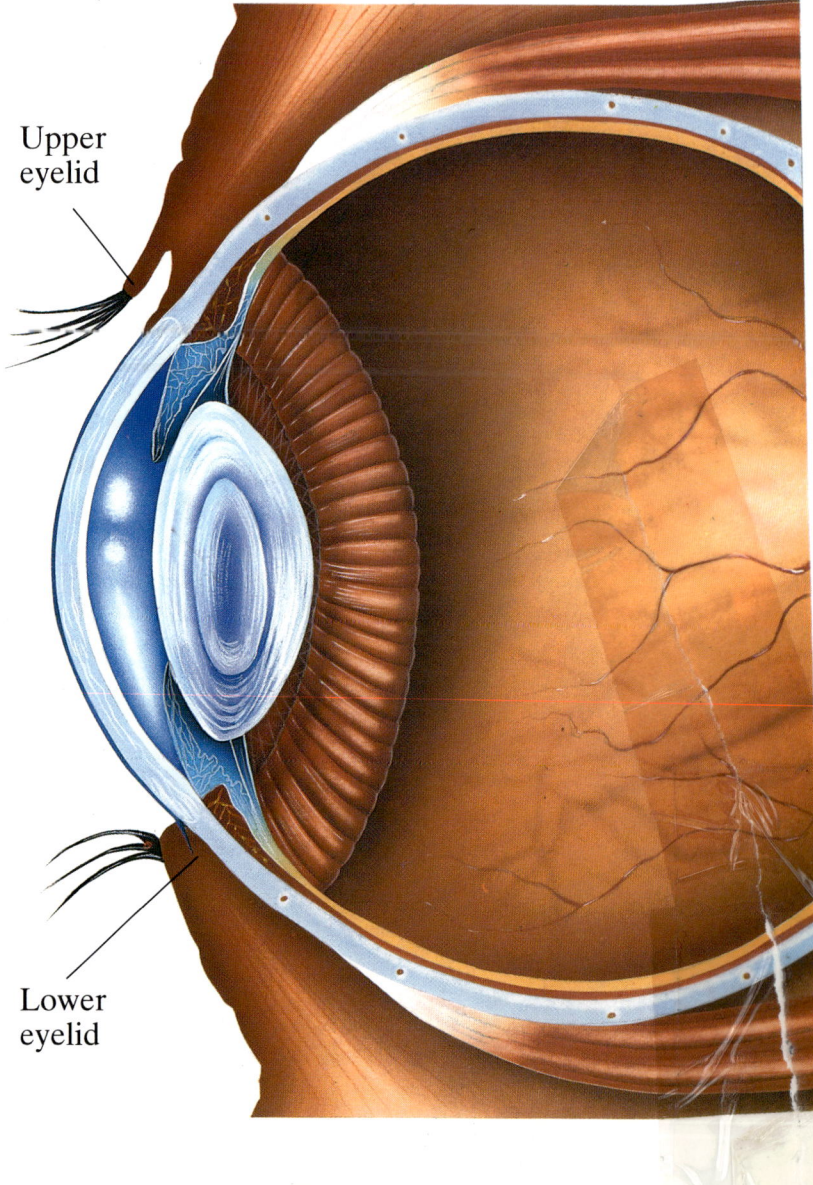

Upper eyelid

Lower eyelid

▲

A hummingbird can hover in the air to take nectar from a flower. It does this by beating its wings very rapidly – its muscles can move far more quickly than any human muscles!

FINDING OUT

Strange messages

Sometimes your muscles produce strange sensations. Stand in a doorway with your arms at your sides. Lift them until the backs of your hands touch the door jambs. Push against them with the backs of your hands and your wrists as hard as you can, while you count slowly to thirty. Step back – and your arms feel as though they are being pulled up towards the ceiling. The brain, through the nerves, has been sending your muscles orders to raise your arms. When you suddenly step back from the doorway and stop pushing, some of the orders are still on their way, so the muscles take a few seconds to receive them.

Tremblers

The more you try to keep the muscles in your arm still, the more they tremble! To demonstrate this, collect three paper clips or pieces of thin wire about 15 centimetres long and a knife, and stand by a table.

Stretch the paper clips out into a V shape, or if you are using pieces of wire bend them in half. Place the paper clips or the wires along the blade of the knife. Stand next to the table and hold the knife in your right hand, with the tips of the wires only just touching the table (don't lean your arm on the table or steady the knife). Try to keep the knife and the wires still ... What happens?

Inside each muscle there are always some fibres which are contracting and others which are relaxing. Each time they change from one state to the other, the muscle quivers slightly. This means that you cannot keep your arm absolutely steady.

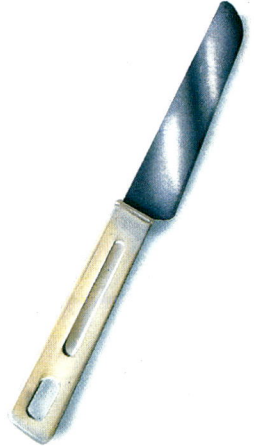

Knife

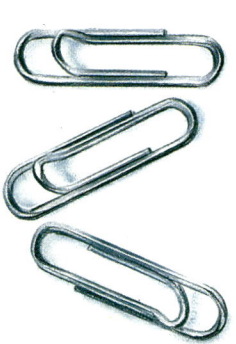

Paper clips

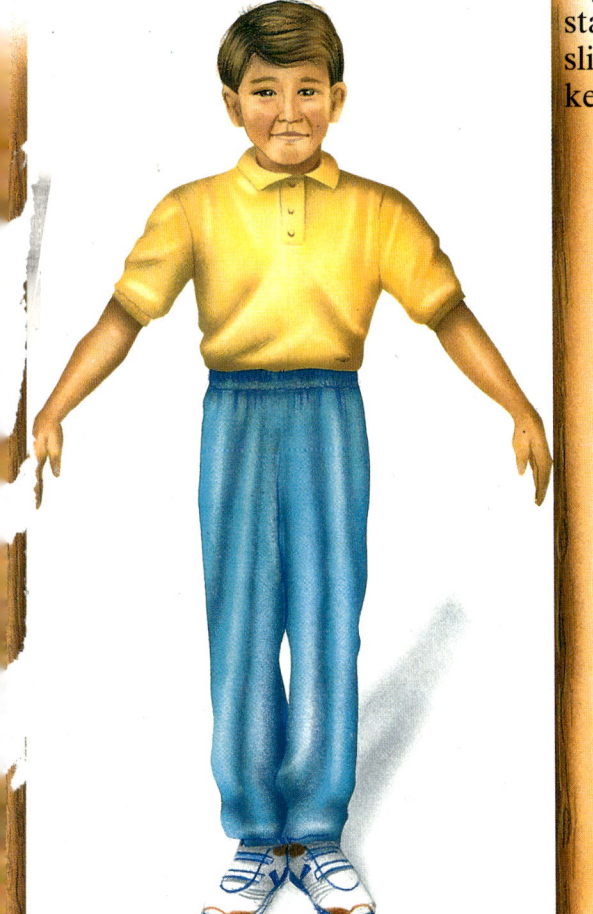

THE MUSCLES

Index and glossary

A

Abdomen 6, 18, 22
The largest cavity in the body, lying below the diaphragm. It is lined with a membrane, and contains the stomach, liver, spleen, pancreas, kidneys, intestines, bladder and some of the reproductive organs.
Achilles tendon 14
Actin 6, 9, 11
A protein found in muscle fibre filaments.
Aerobic metabolism 10, 11
The process in which oxygen and glucose combine in the cell to produce energy.
Anaerobic metabolism 10, 11
The process in which energy is produced from glucose or glycogen in the cell without oxygen.
Ankle 12
Anus 20, 21
The opening of the lower end of the rectum, controlled by circular sphincter muscles, through which faeces leave the body.
Arm 8, 12, 14-16, 18, 19
Arteries 22, 23
The pulmonary artery takes blood from the heart to the lungs; all other arteries carry freshly oxygenated blood from the heart around the rest of the body.
Arterioles 22
Small arteries that join main arteries to capillaries.
Atrium 24, 25
One of the two upper chambers of the heart. The plural is atria.
Auricle 24
Another name for atrium.

B

Blood supply 10, 22-26
Blood vessels 6, 9, 11, 22-25
Bolus 20
A small, rounded lump of chewed food.
Bone 4, 6, 8, 12, 16
Brain 4, 6, 7, 9, 22
Breastbone 18

Breathing 4, 8, 18
Buttock 13, 14, 15

C

Caecum 21
Calf 14
Capillaries 22
Tiny, thin-walled blood vessels which connect arterioles to veins, and form a network through which food, oxygen and other substances can be exchanged between the blood and the tissues.
Carbohydrate 21, 26
Substance obtained from our food which is converted during digestion into glucose.
Carbon dioxide 10, 11, 22, 24, 25
A gas which forms as a waste product during the body's processes, and which is carried by the blood to the lungs, from which it is breathed out.
Cardia 21
Cardiac muscle 4-7, 22, 24
The special muscle tissue from which the heart is formed.
Cartilage 12, 16
Tough, flexible material that makes up part of the skeleton and also the ear flap and part of the nose.
Cells, muscle *see* Fibres, muscle
Cereals 26
Chest 6, 18, 19, 24
The upper part of the body's trunk, also known as the thorax, lying above the diaphragm. The bones of the chest cage enclose a cavity containing the lungs and heart and through which passes the upper part of the digestive tract.
Chewing 16
Chocolate 26
Chyme 20
The mixture of partly digested food and gastric juices passed from the stomach to the duodenum.
Circulation *see* Pulmonary circulation, systemic circulation
Clavicle 12
Another name for the collarbone.

Collarbone 12
Colon 12

D

Deltoid 5, 14
Dermis 17
Diaphragm 18
A dome-shaped sheet of muscle that separates the chest cavity from the abdomen below.
Diet 26
Digestion 4, 20, 23
The process by which our food is broken down into nutrients that can be absorbed and used by the body's cells.
Digestive tract 4, 20, 21
A long tube running through the body from the mouth to the anus, and associated organs, in which digestion takes place.

E

Eating 26
Eggs 26
Elbow 12
Enzymes 21
Protein products of our cells that take part in chemical changes in the body while remaining unchanged themselves.
Epidermis 17
Exercise 8, 11, 24, 26, 27
Expression, facial 16
Eye 4, 16, 17

F

Face 8, 16, 17
Fat 21, 26
Femur 12
The thighbone.
Fibre (dietary) 26
Fibre *see* muscle fibre
Filaments 6, 9, 11, 24
Threadlike structures; filaments of the proteins actin and myosin are found in muscle fibres.
Fingers 14
Fish 26
Food 20, 26
Foot 13, 14
Fruit 26

INDEX AND GLOSSARY

G
Glucose 6, 10, 11, 26
A form of sugar produced by the breaking down of carbohydrates in our food, which supplies energy to the body.
Glycogen 10, 11
The form in which glucose is stored in the liver and muscles. When energy is needed, glycogen is quickly converted back into glucose.
Gymnasts 27

H
Hand 4, 14, 15
Head 16
Heart 4, 10, 18, 22-26
The muscular organ, situated in the chest, which pumps blood round the body and through the lungs, maintaining the body's circulation.
Hiccups 18
Involuntary and painful spasms of the diaphragm.
Hip 12, 14, 15
Hormones 4, 20, 22
Chemicals produced by glands and specialized cells in the body, which control body processes. They are carried round in the blood.
Humerus 12
The bone of the upper arm.

I, J, K
Intestines 6, 18, 21
The tubes that make up the lower part of the digestive tract.
Involuntary muscle 4-7, 20-23
Muscle made up of smooth fibres, not under our conscious control. Also called smooth muscle.
Jaw 18
Joints 8, 9, 12
Knee 12-14
Kneecap 12
Small, triangular bone, contained in the tendon passing over the knee and unattached to any other bone, also known as the patella.

L
Lactic acid 10, 11
A waste product produced in muscles as a result of anaerobic metabolism.
Leg 13-15, 22
Ligament 12
A band of strong, fibrous tissue used to hold bones in place.
Lipase 21
An enzyme taking part in digestion.
Lips 16
Lungs 10, 18, 22-26
Two large organs found in the chest, inside the rib cage. They breathe in air, and exchange its oxygen for the waste-product carbon dioxide carried in the blood. They then breathe out the carbon dioxide.

M
Meat 26
Membrane 6
A thin layer of tissue that covers or contains part of the body.
Menisci 12
Two halfmoon-shaped discs of fibrous cartilage found in the knee.
Milk 26
Minerals 26
Chemical elements, some of which are essential to healthy live.
Mitochondria 6
Muscle fibre 4-7, 9-11, 26
The name commonly used for a muscle cell.
Muscles
    adductor 14, 15
    anal sphincters 20, 21
    antagonistic 14
    biceps 5, 8, 14, 15
    biceps femoris 5, 14, 15
    buccinator 16
    deltoid 4, 5, 14, 15, 19
    extensors 5, 8, 14, 15
    flexors 5, 8, 14, 15
    gastrocnemius 5, 14, 15
    gluteus 5, 13, 15
    hamstrings 14
    inferior oblique 17
    inferior rectus 17
    intercostal 18, 19
    lateral rectus 17
    latissimus dorsi
    masseter 16
    medial rectus 17
    oblique 5, 18, 19
    occipitofrontalis 17
    occipitus 5, 16
    orbicularis oculi 17
    orbicularis oris 17
    pectoral 4, 14, 18, 19
    peroneus longis 5
    pronator 14
    pyloric sphincter 20, 21
    quadriceps 5, 12-15
    rectus abdominis 5, 18, 19
    rectus femoris 5, 14, 15
    rhomboid major 5
    sartorius 5, 15
    serratus 5, 16, 18, 19
    soleus 5, 14, 15
    sternomastoid 16, 17
    superior oblique 17
    superior rectus 17
    supinator 14
    temporalis 16
    tibialis anterior 5
    trapezius 5, 16, 19
    triceps 5, 8, 12, 14, 15
    vastus intermedius 14, 15
    vastus lateralis 14, 15
    vastus medialis 14, 15
    zygomaticus 17
    see also cardiac muscle, involuntary muscle, voluntary muscle
Myosin 6, 9, 11
A protein found in filaments in the muscle fibre.

N
Neck 12, 16
Nerves 4, 6, 9
Nutrients 6, 9, 20, 23, 24, 26
Substances derived from food that are used to build new cells and tissues or are used to provide the body with energy.

O
Oesophagus 4, 20, 21
The muscular tube down which food travels from the pharynx to the stomach.
Oxygen 6, 9-11, 22-26
A gas essential to life, which is absorbed through the lungs and carried by the blood to all the body's tissues, where it is used to 'burn' food to release energy.

P
Pancreas 21
Patella 12
Another name for the kneecap.

Pelvis 18
A bony cavity at the base of the abdomen.
Pepsin 21
An enzyme taking part in digestion.
Peristaltic waves 4, 20, 21
Contractions of the muscles round the oesophagus, stomach and intestines that squeeze along their contents.
Pharynx 4
Proteins 21, 26
Substances obtained from our food that are essential for the body's growth and maintenance.
Pulmonary artery 22
Pulmonary circulation 22-26
Circulation in which blood from the veins is pumped from the right side of the heart to the lungs, where it gives up carbon dioxide and picks up fresh oxygen. It goes back to the left side of the heart.
Pulmonary vein 22

R
Rectum 21
Ribs 18, 19

S
Sarcolemma 6, 9
The outer membrane of the muscle cell.
Scapula 12
Another name for the shoulderblade.
Shin 12
Shoulder 4, 12, 15, 16, 18, 19
Skeletal muscle *see* Voluntary muscle
Skeleton 6, 12
Skin 8, 16, 17
Skull 12
Smooth muscle *see* Involuntary muscle
Sphincter 6, 20
A ring-shaped muscle that closes an opening in the body.
Spine 12
Sports 27
Stomach 4, 6, 18, 20, 21
A major organ of digestion, at the lower end of the oesophagus. Its muscular walls churn the food around to break it down and mix it with the gastric juices.
Striated muscle *see* Voluntary muscle
Systemic circulation 23-25
Circulation in which freshly oxygenated blood is pumped from the left side of the heart round the body. It releases oxygen and nutrients, picks up waste and returns to the right side of the heart.

T
Teeth 16
Temperature 22
Tendon 8, 12
Strong fibrous tissue that attaches muscle to bone.
Thigh 13-15
Thorax 6, 8, 19, 24
Another name for the chest.
Thumb 14
Tibia 12
The larger bone in the lower part of the leg.
Toes 13, 14
Tongue 20
Trunk (of body) 14, 18

V
Vegetables 26
Veins 22
Blood vessels that carry stale blood from the body back to the heart.
Ventricles 24, 25
The two lower chambers of the heart.
Vitamins 26
Substances obtained from food essential to the healthy functioning of the body.
Voluntary muscle 4-19
Muscle made up of striated (striped) fibre, which can be consciously controlled.

W
Water 10, 26
Wrist 12